Recent Advances in

Otolaryngology 8

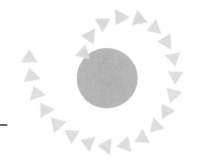

Recent Advances in

Otolaryngology 8

Edited by

David Moffat BSc MA FRCS

Consultant in Otoneurological and Skull Base Surgery,
Addenbrooke's Hospital, Cambridge, UK

James Keir MRCS DOHNS

Specialist Registrar in Otolaryngology, Royal Liverpool
Children's Hospital, Alder Hey, Liverpool, UK

Holger Sudhoff MD PhD

Professor and Chairman, Department of
Otorhinolaryngology, Head and Neck Surgery,
Bielefeld Academic Teaching Hospital,
Bielefeld, Germany

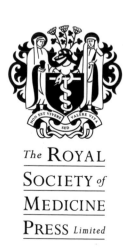

The ROYAL
SOCIETY *of*
MEDICINE
PRESS *Limited*

Published by the Royal Society of Medicine Press Ltd
1 Wimpole Street, London W1G 0AE, UK
Tel: +44 (0)20 7290 2921
Fax: +44 (0)20 7290 2929
Email: publishing@rsm.ac.uk
Website: www.rsmpress.co.uk

British Library Cataloguing in Publication Data
A catalogue record for this book is available from the British Library
ISBN 978–1–85315–711–0

Distribution in Europe and Rest of World:

Marston Book Services Ltd
PO Box 269, Abingdon
Oxon OX14 4YN, UK
Tel: +44 (0)1235 465500
Fax: +44 (0)1235 465555
Email: direct.order@marston.co.uk

Distribution in the USA and Canada:

Royal Society of Medicine Press Ltd
c/o BookMasters Inc
30 Amberwood Parkway
Ashland, OH 44805, USA
Tel: +1 800 247 6553/+1 800 266 5564
Fax: +1 419 281 6883
Email: order@bookmasters.com

Distribution in Australia and New Zealand:

Elsevier Australia
30–52 Smidmore Street
Marrickville NSW 2204, Australia
Tel: +61 2 9517 8999
Fax: +61 2 9517 2249
Email: service@elsevier.com.au

Editorial services and typesetting by BA & GM Haddock, Ford, Midlothian, UK

Printed in India by Replika Press

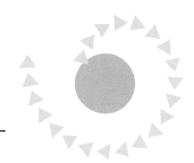

Contents

OTOLOGY

1. MRI of cholesteatoma   1
   Bert De Foer, Jean-Philippe Vercruysse, Erwin Offeciers, Jan W. Casselman

2. Bacterial biofilm infections in otology   21
   Richard A. Chole, Osarenoma Olomu, Eric W. Wang

3. Auditory midbrain implant: experimental and clinical results   33
   Thomas Lenarz, Hubert H. Lim, Minoo Lenarz

4. Bilateral cochlear implantation   55
   Joachim Müller

5. Squamous cell carcinoma of the temporal bone: current evidence for radiotherapy alone and surgery with postoperative radiotherapy   63
   David A. Moffat, Tim Price

6. Reflux and otitis media with effusion   79
   Holger Sudhoff, Désirée Garten, Sören Schreiber

HEAD AND NECK

7. Proteomics and genomics of head and neck squamous cell carcinoma   95
   James Keir, Helen Beer, Terry Jones

8. Vaccines and immunotherapy in head and neck cancer   111
   David F. Hall, William B. Coman

9. Chemoradiotherapy for head and neck cancer   121
   Judith A. Christian, Matthew Griffin, Patrick J. Bradley

RHINOLOGY

10. Image-guided surgery in paranasal sinus and skull base surgery   137
    Anshul Sama, Nick S. Jones

11. Questioning the prevalence of chronic rhinosinusitis   147
    Anu Daudia, Nick S. Jones

PAEDIATRICS

12. New treatments in recurrent respiratory papillomatosis   155
    James Keir, Ray Clarke

Index   171

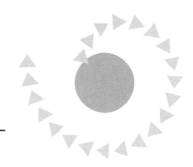

Contributors

Helen Beer MRCS(Ed)
Specialist Registrar in Otolaryngology, Countess of Chester Hospital, Chester, UK

Patrick J. Bradley MBA FRCS
Professor and Consultant in Head and Neck Oncologic Surgery, Department of Otolaryngology,
Nottingham University Hospitals, Queen's Medical Centre Campus, Nottingham, UK

Jan W. Casselman MD PhD
Department of Radiology, Sint-Augustinus Hospital, Wilrijk (Antwerp), Belgium and
Department of Radiology, AZ Sint-Jan AV, Brugge, Belgium

Richard A. Chole MD PhD
Lindburg Professor and Chairman, Department of Otolaryngology, School of Medicine,
Washington University in St Louis, St Louis, Missouri, USA

Judith A. Christian MRCP FRCR MD
Consultant Clinical Oncologist, Department of Oncology, Nottingham University Hospitals,
City Hospital Campus, Nottingham, UK

Ray Clarke BSc DCH FRCS FRCS(ORL)
Consultant in Otolaryngology, Royal Liverpool Children's Hospital, Alder Hey, Liverpool, UK

William B. Coman AM MD
Professor in Otolaryngology, Department of Otolaryngology, Head and Neck Surgery, The
Princess Alexandra Hospital and University of Queensland, Woolloongabba, Queensland,
Australia

Anu Daudia FRCS
Specialist Registrar in Otolaryngology, Department of Otolaryngology, Head and Neck Surgery,
Queen's Medical Centre, University of Nottingham, Nottingham, UK

Bert De Foer MD
Department of Radiology, Sint-Augustinus Hospital, Wilrijk (Antwerp), Belgium

Désirée Garten
Physician Scientist, Institut für Physiologie der Ruhr-Universität Bochum, Germany

Matthew Griffin MRCP FRCR
Specialist Registrar in Oncology, Department of Oncology, Nottingham University Hospitals,
City Hospital Campus, Nottingham, UK

David F. Hall BSc(Hons)(NSW) MBBS(Qld)
ENT Registrar, Department of Otolaryngology, Head and Neck Cancer Unit, The Princess
Alexandra Hospital, Woolloongabba, Queensland, Australia

Nick S. Jones MD FRCS
Professor of Otolaryngology, Department of Otolaryngology, Head and Neck Surgery, Queen's
Medical Centre, University of Nottingham, Nottingham, UK

Terry Jones BSc(Hons) MD FRCS
Senior Lecturer and Honorary Consultant in Head and Neck Cancer Surgery / Otolaryngology,
School of Cancer Studies, University of Liverpool, Liverpool, UK

James Keir MRCS DOHNS
Specialist Registrar in Otolaryngology, Royal Liverpool Children's Hospital, Alder Hey,
Liverpool, UK

Minoo Lenarz MD
Otolaryngologist and Neck Surgeon, Assistant Professor in the Otolaryngology
Department, Medical University of Hannover, Hannover, Germany

Thomas Lenarz MD PhD
Professor and Director of the Otolaryngology Department, Medical University of Hannover,
Hannover, Germany

Hubert H. Lim PhD
Postdoctoral Research Scientist, Department of Otorhinolaryngology, Hannover Medical
University, Hannover, Germany; and Engineering Consultant, Cochlear Ltd, Lane Cove,
Australia

David A. Moffat BSc MA FRCS
Consultant in Otoneurological and Skull Base Surgery, Addenbrooke's Hospital, Cambridge, UK

Joachim Müller MD PhD
Assistant Professor, Department of Otolaryngology, Head and Neck Surgery at the University of
Würzburg, Germany; Schwerpunkt Cochlea Implantate und Hörprothetik — Internationales
Referenzzentrum; Klinik und Poliklinik für Hals-, Nasen- und Ohrenkranke der Universität,
Würzburg, Germany

Erwin Offeciers MD PhD
University Department of ENT, Sint-Augustinus Hospital, Wilrijk (Antwerp), Belgium

Osarenoma Olomu MD
Department of Otolaryngology, School of Medicine, Washington University in St Louis, St Louis,
Missouri, USA

Tim Price BSc DLO FRCS (ORL HNS)
Consultant ENT Surgeon, Dorset County Hospital, Dorchester, UK

Anshul Sama FRCS
Consultant in Otorhinolaryngology, Department of Otorhinolaryngology, Head and Neck
Surgery, Queen's Medical Centre, Nottingham University Hospital, Nottingham, UK

Sören Schreiber MD PhD
Associate Professor, Institut für Physiologie der Ruhr-Universität Bochum, Germany

Holger Sudhoff MD PhD
Professor, Chairman and Medical Director, Department of Otorhinolaryngology, Head and Neck
Surgery, Bielefeld Academic Teaching Hospital, Affiliated to Münster University, Bielefeld,
Germany

Jean-Philippe Vercruysse MD
University Department of ENT, Sint-Augustinus Hospital, Wilrijk (Antwerp), Belgium

Eric W. Wang MD
Department of Otolaryngology, School of Medicine, Washington University in St Louis, St
Louis, Missouri, USA

Bert De Foer Jean-Philippe Vercruysse
Erwin Offeciers Jan W. Casselman

MRI of cholesteatoma

Although computed tomography (CT) is still the method of choice for the evaluation of a primary acquired or congenital middle ear cholesteatoma, magnetic resonance imaging (MRI) is gaining growing importance. In acquired or congenital middle ear cholesteatoma, MRI including late post-gadolinium T1-weighted and non-echo planar diffusion-weighted sequences are superior in the discrimination of the cholesteatoma from surrounding inflammation and in the description of possible associated complications. In the postoperative follow-up of cholesteatoma, MRI has been proven to be superior to CT in the detection of residual or recurrent cholesteatoma.

Cholesteatoma should be divided upon its origin into acquired and congenital cholesteatoma.[1] Congenital cholesteatoma commonly involves extradural structures predominantly including the middle ear cavity and mastoid but also involving other portions of the petrous bone including the petrous apex and external auditory canal. It originates at the time of closure of the neural tube when ectoderm gets trapped inside the temporal bone. This should be discriminated from another congenital entity originating at this point: the epidermoid cyst or epidermoid tumour, when

Bert De Foer MD (for correspondence)
Radiologist, Department of Radiology, Sint-Augustinus Hospital, Oosterveldlaan 24, 2610 Wilrijk (Antwerp), Belgium
E-mail: bert.defoer@GZA.be

Jean-Philippe Vercruysse MD
ENT Surgeon and Doctoral Fellow, University Department of ENT, Sint-Augustinus Hospital, Oosterveldlaan 24, 2610 Wilrijk (Antwerp), Belgium

Erwin Offeciers MD PhD
ENT Surgeon, Head of Department, University Department of ENT, Sint-Augustinus Hospital, Oosterveldlaan 24, 2610 Wilrijk (Antwerp), Belgium

Jan W. Casselman MD PhD
Radiologist, Head of Department, Department of Radiology, AZ Sint-Jan AV, Ruddershove 10, 8000 Brugge, Belgium; and Consultant at Department of Radiology, Sint-Augustinus Hospital, Oosterveldlaan 24, 2610 Wilrijk (Antwerp), Belgium

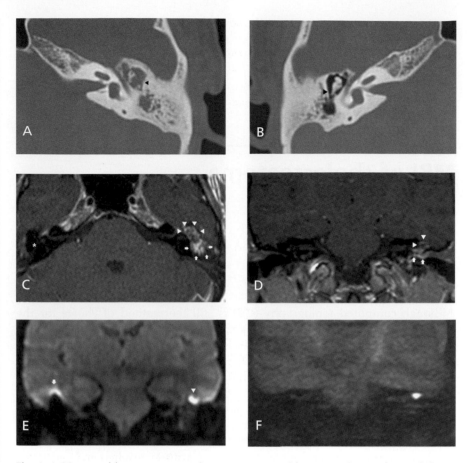

Fig. 1 A 39-year-old woman presenting at otoscopy with a retraction pocket and signs of associated infection and inflammation. CT already demonstrated signs of a cholesteatoma by showing erosion of incus corpus and short process. MRI performed using echoplanar diffusion-weighted and non-echoplanar diffusion-weighted sequences clearly shows the advantages of non-echoplanar diffusion-weighted over echoplanar diffusion-weighted sequences in demonstrating the cholesteatoma.
(A) Axial CT image on the left side, at the level of the tympanic segment of the facial nerve showing a complete erosion of the incus corpus and short process (arrowhead) by an associated soft tissue mass filling up the entire epitympanic cavity.
(B) Axial CT image on the right side (same level as [A]) showing a normal ossicular chain. Note the completely normal aspect of the incus corpus and short process (arrowhead) and the well-aerated middle-ear cavity.
(C) Axial late post-gadolinium T1-weighted MR image (same level as [A,B]) shows the normal signal void (black or hypo-intense signal) of the normal aerated antrum on the right side (asterisk). On the left side, the cholesteatoma can be seen as an approximately 1 cm large hypo-intense non-enhancing lesion in the epitympanum and antrum (arrowheads). Note the surrounding enhancing inflammation presenting as hyperintense material filling the antrum and mastoid (arrows).
(D) Coronal late post-gadolinium T1-weighted MR image at the level of the internal auditory canal. The cholesteatoma is demonstrated as a rather small nodular hypo-intense non-enhancing lesion in the antrum, almost immediately under the tegmen (arrowheads). Note the extensive surrounding inflammation presenting as hyperintense enhancing soft tissue (arrows).
(E) Coronal echoplanar diffusion-weighted imaging through both temporal bones. On the right side, the characteristic curvilinear artefact is noted at the interface temporal lobe temporal bone (arrow). On the left side, a somewhat nodular hyperintense signal is seen underneath the temporal lobe (arrowhead). Due to the frequent susceptibility artefact, differentiation with a cholesteatoma remains difficult (compare to [F]),

ectodermal tissue gets entrapped intradurally instead of extradurally in the temporal bone. Essentially, congenital cholesteatoma and epidermoid tumour are congenital lesions and are histologically the same.

Lesions can thus be found in any part of the temporal bone pyramid.[2] By definition, congenital cholesteatoma presents itself behind an intact tympanic membrane without any signs of infection. In the middle ear, the majority of lesions arise in the anterior mesotympanum or posterior epitympanum.[3]

Acquired cholesteatoma often originates from a posterosuperior retraction pocket of the tympanic membrane (pars flaccida cholesteatoma). A less frequent variant originates at the lower part of the tympanic membrane (pars tensa cholesteatoma).[1,4] Acquired pars flaccida cholesteatoma originates out of retractions of the tympanic membrane, progressively evolving into Prussak's space. Due to its expansion, the cholesteatoma starts eroding surrounding structures such as the bony spur of the scutum and the ossicular chain; mainly the head of the malleus and the long process and body of the incus.[1,4] Growing further, the cholesteatoma invades the antrum and mastoid space, eroding additional structures of the middle ear cavity such as the bony cover over the second segment of the facial canal, the tegmen of the middle ear and the bony delineation of the lateral semicircular canal.[1,4]

Cholesteatoma is mainly operated on using canal-wall-up (CWU) techniques implying the preservation of the external auditory canal wall and its consequent benefits.[5,6] This leads to an increased risk of leaving residual cholesteatoma behind in comparison with canal-wall-down (CWD) techniques.[5-7] The surgical strategy in CWU techniques, however, necessitates the need to perform second-stage surgery in order to detect residual cholesteatoma. Usually, these residual cholesteatoma are very small pearls.[7]

This should be differentiated from the recurrent cholesteatoma which develops out of a new posterosuperior retraction pocket.[7] Recurrent cholesteatoma are often detected during clinical follow-up by micro-otoscopical investigation.

In order to diminish the rate of recurrent cholesteatoma, mastoid and epitympanic obliteration techniques have been advocated. Here, the mastoid and epitympanic cavity are sealed off from the middle ear space by means of sculpted cortical bone chips and subsequently the remainder of the mastoid and epitympanum is obliterated with bone paste. As a result of this primary bony obliteration technique (PBOT), the percentage of recurrence may drop from 36% in adults and 67% in children after a CWU procedure to a few percent in PBOT.[8-10]

CT IMAGING OF CHOLESTEATOMA

High-resolution CT of the temporal bone is still the imaging modality of choice to evaluate the extension of a suspected acquired middle ear cholesteatoma,

Fig. 1 *(continued)*
(F) Coronal non-echoplanar diffusion-weighted sequence (single shot turbo spin echo diffusion-weighted image) B1000 image (same level as [E]). The cholesteatoma is seen as a small hyperintense nodular lesion underneath the left temporal lobe. Note the clear visualisation of the cholesteatoma and the complete absence of any susceptibility artefact. Compared to (E), this image demonstrates the superiority of non-echoplanar diffusion-weighted sequences over echoplanar diffusion-weighted sequences in the detection of middle ear cholesteatoma. Note that the sequence only demonstrates the cholesteatoma.

prior to eventual surgery. High-resolution CT of the temporal bone is able to show the sometimes subtle details of a small cholesteatoma.[1,4]

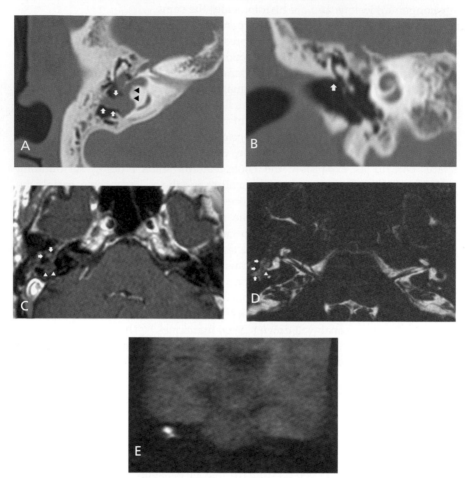

Fig. 2 A 53-year-old woman with severe conductive hearing loss. Otoscopy showed an intact tympanic membrane.

(A) Axial CT image of the right ear at the level of the lateral semicircular canal showing a large soft tissue lesion (arrows) nearly completely filling up the antrum and mastoid. There is subtle erosion of the incus body and short process. The soft tissue mass invades the lateral semicircular canal (arrowheads).

(B) Coronal CT reformation at the level of the cochlea showing an intact scutum (arrow). Note the well aerated aspect of Prussak's space and intact aspect of the pars flaccida of the tympanic membrane (arrow). There is no suggestion on CT of an acquired pars flaccida cholesteatoma.

(C) Axial late post-gadolinium T1-weighted MR image at the level of the internal auditory canal and vestibule showing the cholesteatoma as a nodular non-enhancing lesion mainly situated in the posterior antrum (arrowheads). There is some associated enhancement in the anterior epitympanic space (arrows). There seems to be no obvious enhancement of the membranous labyrinth.

(D) Axial 0.4 mm thick slice out of a 3-D TSE T2-weighted sequence showing the cholesteatoma as an intermediate signal intensity lesion (arrows) invading the lateral semicircular canal (arrowhead). The signal inside the membranous labyrinth on the right side is comparable to the signal on the normal left side.

(E) Coronal SS TSE diffusion-weighted sequence demonstrates a hyperintense lesion in the right middle ear, confirming the diagnosis of a middle ear cholesteatoma. Again, only the cholesteatoma is highlighted by the sequence.

The more common pars flaccida cholesteatoma starts with a retraction pocket into Prussak's space. This retraction pocket is best evaluated at otoscopy and can be seen on coronal CT scans or reformations. Very often, an associated nodular soft tissue lesion can be found in Prussak's space. Erosion caused by the pars flaccida cholesteatoma usually starts at the lateral epitympanic recessus with erosion of the scutum and the lateral epitympanic wall (Fig. 1).

It can erode the malleus head, the corpus and short process of the incus as well as the long process. These often subtle details can best be seen when comparing both ears on CT scan. In case of further growth, the cholesteatoma grows into the antrum and further into the mastoid cavity. The cholesteatoma can also erode the tegmen which is best evaluated in the coronal plane. Direct coronal images are preferred over coronal reconstruction of a spiral scan as the tegmen can be better delineated on direct coronal images. The bony delineation of the lateral semicircular canal should always be examined carefully in order to exclude fistulisation to the lateral semicircular canal. Special attention should be paid to the tympanic or second segment of the facial nerve canal as this is also prone to erosion by a middle-ear cholesteatoma.[1,4]

It should be noted that bony erosion can also be seen in cases of non-cholesteatomatous disease. Ossicular chain erosions are rather rare in case of non-cholesteatomatous middle ear disease, but are known to occur and will predominantly erode the incus long process and lenticular process, followed by the stapes head. The malleus and incus body are much less vulnerable to this erosion, which is believed to take place under release of substances by mononuclear inflammatory cells and osteocytes or osteoclasts.[11]

Congenital cholesteatoma can originate in every part of the temporal bone pyramid. In cases of the more frequent middle ear presentation, one usually can find a small nodular soft tissue density located in the anterosuperior part of the mesotympanum or in the posterior epitympanum.[3] This nodular soft tissue is associated with an intact tympanic membrane without any soft tissues in Prussak's space. However, congenital cholesteatoma in the middle ear can present as an aspecific and sometimes large middle ear soft tissue mass. It can also erode the ossicular chain. Invasion into the membranous labyrinth is most frequent at the level of the lateral semicircular canal (Fig. 2). Another frequent location of combined middle ear and temporal bone pyramid congenital cholesteatoma is the region of the geniculate ganglion of the facial nerve.[1,3]

In the case of petrous bone apex presentation, it usually presents as a sharply delineated punched-out lesion associated to a soft tissue mass. The sharp and regular delineation of congenital cholesteatoma in the temporal bone pyramid is its most important characteristic in the differential diagnosis with other lesions such as metastasis or glomus tumour. Depending on its position, it may invade essential parts of the membranous labyrinth, such as the cochlea, the vestibule and semicircular canals as well as all the segments of the facial canal (Fig. 3).[1,4]

MRI OF CHOLESTEATOMA

MRI has the capability of multiplanar imaging and has a superior soft tissue differentiation. It was noted in the early 1990s that MRI was able to differentiate cholesteatoma from inflammatory tissue using gadolinium enhanced T1-weighted sequences.[12] This is based upon the observation that cholesteatoma is, by definition, an avascular tissue and does not enhance after

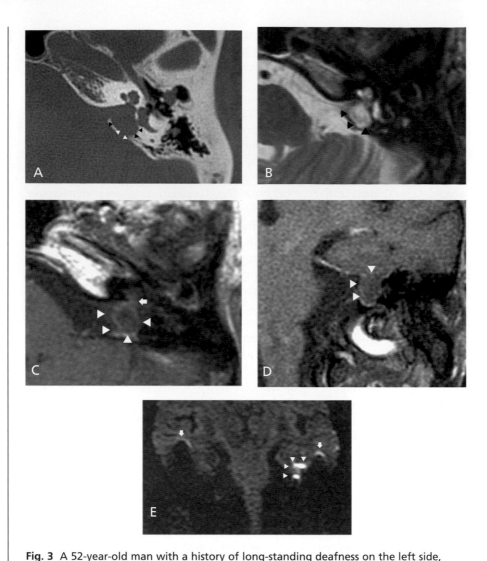

Fig. 3 A 52-year-old man with a history of long-standing deafness on the left side, presenting with a sudden, severe and persistent facial palsy. Presumed diagnosis on CT and MRI was a congenital cholesteatoma. Surgery confirmed a congenital cholesteatoma. Note the hyperintense aspect of the congenital cholesteatoma on echoplanar diffusion-weighted and the distorted aspect of the lesion and the artefact at the interface between temporal lobe and temporal bone. These imaging findings are very characteristic for echoplanar diffusion-weighted sequences.

(A) Axial CT scan of the temporal bone at the level of the internal auditory canal shows a sharply delineated hypodense lesion situated posterior to the internal auditory canal (arrowheads). The delineation is lost between the lesion and the internal auditory canal. The sharp delineation of the lesion and the absence of a moth-eaten aspect of the adjacent bone makes the diagnosis of a metastatic lesion less probable.

(B) Axial T2-weighted MR image of the skull (same level as [A]) shows a nodular intense lesion posterior to the internal auditory canal (arrowhead). Lesion with aspecific signal intensity on this MRI of the head.

(C) Axial post-gadolinium T1-weighted image of the temporal bone (same level as [A,B]) clearly shows the centrally non-enhancing hypo-intense lesion of the left temporal bone (arrowheads). The lesion cannot be delineated from the internal auditory canal suggestive of invasion. Note the thin enhancing matrix around the non-enhancing keratin in the cholesteatoma. There seems to be also some enhancement in the modiolus of the cochlea (arrow), suggestive of invasion.

intravenous (i.v.) gadolinium (Gd) contrary to the enhancing inflammatory tissue. On T2-weighted images, cholesteatoma shows an intermediate hyperintensity, clearly lower than the intensity of accumulated fluid and associated inflammation. The signal intensity of a cholesteatoma looks somewhat similar to that of the grey matter of brain on T2-weighted MRI (Figs 4 and 5).

Recent papers have described aspects of cholesteatoma on diffusion-weighted MRI sequences.[13,14] The mechanism of diffusion-weighted-MRI is based on the Brownian motion of water molecules in tissue and, more importantly, on the hindrances/facilitations of the water molecule movements in various types of tissue. In order to make an MRI sequence sensitive to the diffusion of water molecules, the sequence is expanded with a diffusion-sensitizing gradient scheme, usually a very fast, single-shot gradient-echo data collecting sequence (echoplanar). The amount of diffusion-sensitizing applied is usually indicated by the b-value. In clinical practice, images are generally acquired with a b-value of 1000 s/mm^2. Diffusion-weighted-MRI is now an established method used routinely for the diagnosis of acute stroke.[15] Extracranial applications of diffusion-weighted MRI are becoming increasingly important.[16]

Fitzek and colleagues[13] were one of the first groups to report that cholesteatoma is hyperintense on echoplanar diffusion-weighted MRI, more specifically on B1000 images. However, echoplanar diffusion-weighted MRI has the major drawback of a low spatial resolution, a higher slice thickness and a major susceptibility artefact at the interface between air and bone. This clearly limits its value for the diagnosis of middle ear cholesteatoma (Fig. 1).[14,17] Very recently, two types of non-echoplanar based diffusion-weighted sequences have been described for the diagnosis of middle ear cholesteatoma.[17,18] These turbo spin echo (TSE) or fast spin echo (FSE) based diffusion-weighted sequences have a higher spatial resolution, generate thinner slices and do not suffer at all from susceptibility artefacts. The single-shot TSE diffusion-weighted sequence uses a 180° radiofrequency refocusing pulse for each measured echo, which explains the reduction of the susceptibility artefact (Fig. 1).[17]

First reports of results in larger series indicate a much higher sensitivity and specificity for the diagnosis of middle-ear cholesteatoma using these non-echoplanar based diffusion-weighted sequences[19] in which cholesteatoma also appears hyperintense on B1000 images.

MRI OF CONGENITAL CHOLESTEATOMA

In congenital cholesteatoma in a middle ear location, a nodular soft tissue lesion is most frequently found in the anterosuperior part of the mesotympanum or in the

---

Fig. 3 *(continued)*
(D) Coronal post-gadolinium T1-weighted image with fat saturation. The cholesteatoma can be seen as a nodular hypo-intense lesion (arrowheads), located very medially into the signal void of the temporal bone underneath the left temporal lobe.
(E) Coronal echoplanar diffusion-weighted B1000 images. On this sequence, the lesion can be noted as a rather bi-nodular (instead of oval) hyperintense lesion (arrowheads). Note that the lesion has a distorted aspect (arrowheads) and that there is a curvilinear interface artefact at the border of the temporal lobe and temporal bone on both sides (arrows). Both features are characteristic of an echoplanar diffusion-weighted sequence. However, as the lesion is quite large, echoplanar diffusion-weighted confirms the diagnosis of a congenital cholesteatoma by showing a definite high signal intensity lesion on B1000 images.

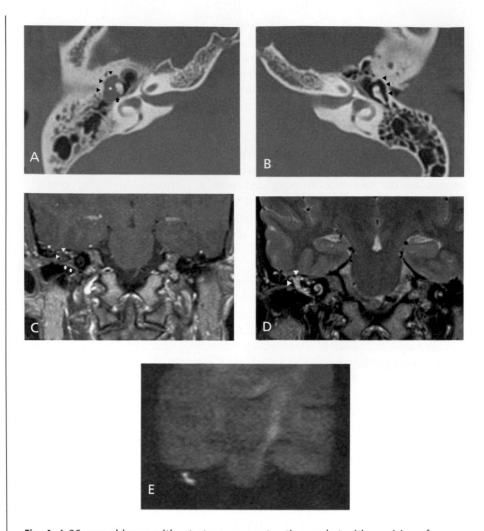

Fig. 4 A 26-year-old man with, at otoscopy, a retraction pocket with suspicion of a cholesteatoma. There was also the clinical suspicion of an associated infection. CT scan shows the signs of the cholesteatoma eroding the ossicular chain. MRI makes it possible to differentiate the cholesteatoma from the surrounding inflammation. Final diagnosis was a middle-ear cholesteatoma originating from a retraction pocket expanding into the antrum and mastoid cavity with surrounding inflammation.
(A) Axial CT image of the right temporal bone at the level of the lateral semicircular canal, showing typical features of middle ear cholesteatoma: erosion of the body and long process of the incus (large arrow) by an associated soft tissue density (asterisk), eroding also the lateral epitympanic wall (arrowheads).
(B) Axial CT image of the left temporal bone (same level as [A]). Note the intact aspect of the ossicular chain, more specifically of the incus body and short process (arrow) and the normal distance between the ossicular chain and lateral epitympanic wall.
(C) Coronal late post-gadolinium T1-weighted MR image at the level of the cochlea clearly showing the non-enhancing cholesteatoma (arrowheads) situated in the antrum with surrounding enhancing inflammation (arrows).
(D) Coronal T2-weighted MR image (same level as [C]) showing the cholesteatoma as an intermediate signal intensity lesion in the right epitympanic cavity (arrowheads).
(E) Coronal non-echoplanar diffusion-weighted sequence (same level as [C]) clearly shows the cholesteatoma in the epitympanic cavity, antrum and mastoid as a small rather bilobar hyperintensity. The clear hyperintensity confirms the diagnosis of a congenital cholesteatoma.

posterior epitympanum (Fig. 2).[1,3] In other temporal bone locations, CT often shows a sharply delineated, hypodense, punched-out, aspecific, soft tissue lesion, which can be located anywhere in the temporal bone pyramid. In the case of a petrous bone apex lesion, the congenital cholesteatoma can invade the membranous labyrinth and facial nerve canal. Usually, such a lesion demonstrates sharp and regular borders contrary to other more aggressive lesions such as metastasis or glomus tumours (Fig. 3).[1,2]

The exact bony delineation of such a lesion can easily be described on CT. MRI is, however, superior in describing the exact location and extension of congenital cholesteatoma in the middle ear or temporal bone pyramid. It is able to demonstrate the relation with other structures of the membranous labyrinth and the facial nerve. Moreover, MRI is able to characterize the lesion with a high degree of confidence (Figs 2 and 3).

If a congenital cholesteatoma is located in the apex of the temporal bone pyramid, differentiating this from an opacified aerated cell in the temporal bone pyramid and a cholesterol granuloma can sometimes be difficult.[20] Cholesterol granuloma, however, displays a clear hyperintensity on T1- and T2-weighted images contrary to cholesteatoma which presents as a lesion with a definite low-signal intensity on T1-weighted images and an intermediate signal on T2-weighted images. An opacified and/or infected aerated cell in the apex of the os petrosum pyramid shows a low signal intensity on T1-weighted MR images and a high signal intensity on T2-weighted MR images making the differential diagnosis with a congenital cholesteatoma complex.[20] Theoretically, signal intensities on T1- as well as on T2-weighted images may vary in time due to the change in water content of the secretions in the opacified cells.[20] In these cases, diffusion-weighted sequences can make the differentiation by showing a high signal intensity lesion on B1000 images in the case of cholesteatoma. One should take into account that the echoplanar diffusion-weighted sequences are very prone to artefacts in the skull base region contrary to the non-echoplanar diffusion-weighted sequences which will clearly show these lesions without artefacts. Moreover, non-echoplanar diffusion-weighted sequences have the capacity of demonstrating even very small congenital cholesteatoma.[19] We consider it important to add a non-echoplanar diffusion-weighted sequence to the standard MRI protocol in cases of MR evaluation of any lytic temporal bone lesion or aspecific middle ear or temporal bone lesion. By doing so, a congenital cholesteatoma will easily be detected without deformation of the region of interest by susceptibility artefacts.

MRI OF ACQUIRED CHOLESTEATOMA

The primary imaging tool for an acquired middle-ear cholesteatoma is high resolution CT of the temporal bone.[1,4] However, in selected cases of an acquired cholesteatoma, MRI has a role. When there is an associated surrounding infection, MRI will be able to delineate the cholesteatoma exactly (Fig. 4).[4,11,17] If there are suspected complications on CT scan, MRI may act as a diagnostic aid (Fig. 5).[17] If a cholesteatoma invades the membranous labyrinth through the lateral semicircular canal, MRI will be able to demonstrate enhancement of the membranous labyrinth on T1-weighted

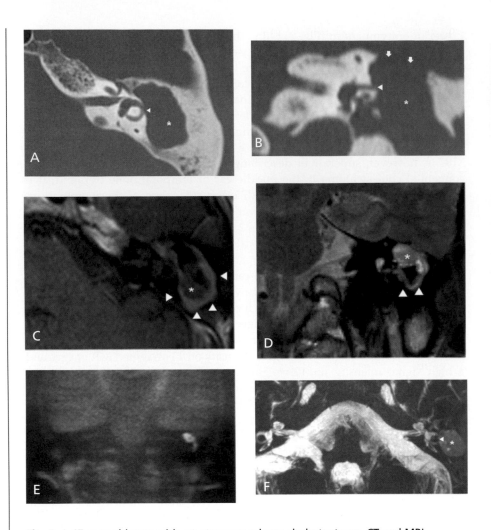

Fig. 5 A 47-year-old man with, at otoscopy, a large cholesteatoma. CT and MRI demonstrate characteristic features of a large middle ear cholesteatoma, with associated complications.

(A) Axial CT scan at the level of the lateral semicircular canal. Completely eroded antrum and mastoid filled with soft tissues (asterisk). No ossicular chain can be delineated. Note the loss of the bony cover over the lateral semicircular canal (arrowhead). Findings are pathognomonic for a large middle ear cholesteatoma with suspicion of fistulisation to the lateral semicircular canal.

(B) Coronal CT reconstruction at the level of the oval window and lateral semicircular canal. There is complete opacification of the middle ear and antrum without any residual ossicular chain (asterisk). The bony delineation over the lateral semicircular canal is lost (arrowhead) suggestive for fistulisation to the lateral semicircular canal. Moreover there is also loss of delineation of the tegmen of the middle ear cavity (arrows) so middle fossa invasion cannot be excluded.

(C) Axial late post-gadolinium T1-weighted MR image at the level of the lateral semicircular canal (same level as [A]). There is enhancement at the periphery of the large antral cavity compatible with matrix and perimatrix of the cholesteatoma (arrowheads). The centrally located hypo-intense soft tissue in the lower part of the large antral cavity is compatible with keratine (asterisk). Compared to the axial CT image in (A), the keratine is partially evacuated due to suction cleaning by the ENT surgeon via the external auditory canal. There seems to be no clear enhancement of the membranous labyrinth. On the coronal image (not shown) no invasion in the middle cranial fossa could be demonstrated.

sequences after gadolinium administration. Signal loss on the heavily T2-weighted sequences (caused by replacement of the fluid by fibrous tissue) can be noted depending on the stage of the associated labyrinthitis (Fig. 5). In the acute phase, enhancement will be noted on T1-weighted images without signal loss on heavily T2-weighted images. In the subacute phase, the enhancement will diminish with subsequent moderate signal loss on heavily T2-weighted sequences. In the chronic phase, no enhancement will be noted with complete signal loss on heavily T2-weighted sequences due to the fibrosis. In case of suspected tegmen disruption on CT, MRI will nicely demonstrate meningeal enhancement in the middle fossa and eventual changes in signal intensity in the adjacent temporal bone on T2-weighted images.

Cholesteatoma displays a hypo-intense aspect on T1-weighted images surrounded by the cholesteatoma matrix and perimatrix, presenting as an enhancing line (Fig. 5). On T2-weighted images, cholesteatoma has an intermediate signal intensity. Usually, even on T2-weighted images, discrimination with surrounding inflammation is possible as inflammation displays a much higher signal intensity.[4,17] On echoplanar diffusion-weighted images, acquired cholesteatoma will (as congenital cholesteatoma) display a clear high-signal intensity on B1000 images.[4,13,14] A recent paper, however, has set the size limit for visualisation of an acquired cholesteatoma at 5 mm due to the above limitations of echoplanar diffusion-weighted MRI, mainly based upon susceptibility artefacts.[14] Thus, any cholesteatoma lesion smaller than 5 mm can be missed, giving the possibility of false-negative lesions. Moreover, a cholesteatoma located in the antrum and mastoid underneath the tegmen can easily be hidden in the curvilinear artefact of the interface of bone and air at the tegmen (Fig. 1).[17] Echoplanar diffusion-weighted MRI can be used to evaluate an acquired middle-ear cholesteatoma taking the limitations into account such as size limit, the distortion of the lesion and the susceptibility artefacts. To date, no false positives have been reported using echoplanar diffusion-weighted sequences.[14]

However, non-echoplanar based diffusion-weighted sequences have been reported to be superior to echoplanar diffusion-weighted sequences demonstrating acquired middle-ear cholesteatoma (Fig. 1).[17,19] These sequences display less artefacts, allow a lower slice thickness and a higher resolution. In a recent study, a specific non-echoplanar based diffusion-weighted sequence (single shot TSE diffusion-weighted) was able to demonstrate acquired middle

---

Fig. 5 *(continued)*
(D) Coronal T2-weighted image at the level of the vestibule showing the partially evacuated cholesteatoma sac (arrowheads) with centrally the intermediate signal of the keratine (asterisk) in the cholesteatoma sac. Compare the signal intensity of the cholesteatoma to the signal intensity of the adjacent temporal lobe. Note the normal signal intensity of the adjacent temporal lobe, excluding invasion.
(E) Coronal non-echoplanar diffusion-weighted image showing a clear hyperintensity under the left temporal lobe. The hyperintensity is caused by the accumulated keratine in the cholesteatoma matrix. Compare to (D).
(F) Maximum intensity projection (or MIP reconstruction) of a 3-D TSE T2-weighted sequence. The cholesteatoma can be seen as a large nodular intermediate signal intensity lesion (asterisk). There is partial loss of delineation of the lateral semicircular canal (arrowhead) with a slight signal loss of the lateral semicircular canal compared to the other side. This signal loss is suggestive of possible onset of fibrosis.

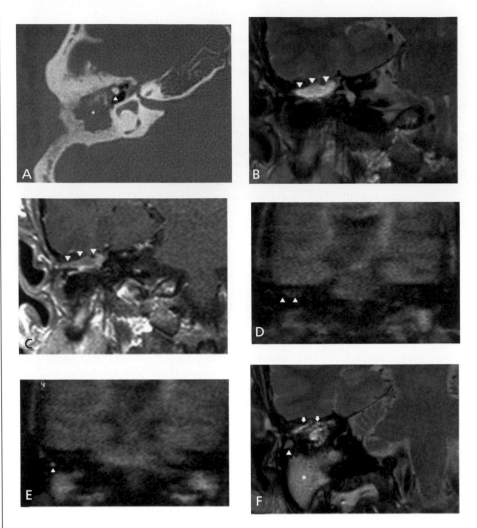

Fig. 6 A 45-year-old man with a history of cholesteatoma surgery on the right side 14 months ago. Follow-up CT and MR examination were performed. Non-echoplanar diffusion-weighted sequence shows a very small residual cholesteatoma pearl located very posteriorly and laterally in the resection cavity. Apart from this very small residual cholesteatoma, the entire resection cavity and middle ear cavity are filled with scar tissue and granulation tissue.

(A) Axial CT scan at the level of the horizontal semicircular canal shows a complete opacification of the mastoidectomy and middle ear cavity (asterisk). Note some bony remnants in the cavity and a part of the head of the malleus (arrowhead). It is impossible to differentiate these soft tissues on CT as scar tissue, granulation tissue, inflammation and cholesteatoma display the same density on CT.

(B) Coronal T2-weighted MR image at the level of the vestibule, superior and lateral semicircular canal. The middle ear and resection cavity are completely filled with homogeneous hyperintense material (arrowheads). Signal intensity is clearly too high to be compatible with cholesteatoma (compare to the signal intensity of the grey matter of the adjacent temporal lobe).

(C) Coronal late post-gadolinium T1-weighted MR image (same level as [B]). Note the complete enhancement of the middle ear and mastoidectomy cavity (arrowheads) excluding any cholesteatoma on this location.

(D) Coronal non-echoplanar diffusion-weighted image: same level (B,C). No clear hyperintensity can be noted in the resection cavity. The soft tissue in the resection cavity displays a moderate to low intensity (arrowheads).

ear cholesteatoma as small as 2 mm.[19] Non-echoplanar diffusion-weighted sequences have two major limitations. Motion artefacts can be a cause of false negatives as in these cases the hyperintense signal on B1000 images is smeared out over multiple pixels, thus causing rather iso-intense signals.[19] Another possible cause of false negatives is the so-called auto-evacuated cholesteatoma.[19] In these cholesteatomas, the content of the retraction pocket is evacuated into the external auditory canal leaving the cholesteatoma matrix behind in its original position in the middle ear and antrum. In these cases, diffusion-weighted sequences (echoplanar as well as non-echoplanar) display no hyperintensity as the keratine in the retraction pocket (responsible for the hyperintense signal on diffusion-weighted sequences) is evacuated. Theoretically, the matrix and perimatrix can be visualized as an enhancing linear structure on T1-weighted post-gadolinium sequences but discrimination is sometimes difficult due to the surrounding inflammation.[19]

MRI OF POSTOPERATIVE CHOLESTEATOMA

The use of canal wall up tympanoplasty frequently necessitates second-look surgery. In a postoperative setting, MRI is clearly superior to CT in the evaluation of the postoperative ear. Despite CT's reported insufficiency for the detection of postoperative cholesteatoma,[23–25] it is still used world-wide in the postoperative evaluation of middle-ear cholesteatoma. Postoperative monitoring for recurrence will probably become one of the most important indications to perform an MRI for cholesteatoma.

CT, however, is not without merit and, in the well-aerated middle ear and postoperative cavity without any associated soft tissue, a high negative predictive value in excluding postoperative residual or recurrent cholesteatoma is seen.[21,22] In nodular-associated soft tissue lesions, CT is able to make the positive diagnosis of a residual or recurrent cholesteatoma.[21,22] However, in the vast majority of cases, the postoperative cavity and middle ear are partially or completely filled with soft tissue densities making differentiation on CT impossible.

Currently, two types of protocols or techniques are used to demonstrate cholesteatoma, especially in the postoperative setting.

Late post-gadolinium T1-weighted imaging

Williams and colleagues[21,22] were the first to report the use of late post-gadolinium T1-weighted sequences for the detection of postoperative residual

---

Fig. 6 (*continued*)
(E) Coronal non-echoplanar diffusion-weighted image posterior in the mastoidectomy cavity. There is a very small nodular hyperintensity visible laterally and posteriorly in the resection cavity (arrowhead). The large nodular moderate intense region caudal to the temporal bone signal void on both sides, is fat in the mastoid tip.
(F) Coronal T2-weighted MR image (same level as [E]). There is a very small, moderately intense nodule lateral and posterior in the mastoidectomy cavity (arrowhead). Note the high signal intensity of fat in the mastoid point (asterisk). The rest of the mastoidectomy cavity is filled with high signal intensity material compatible (arrows) with scar tissue and granulation tissue. The very small, moderately intense nodule corresponds to the visualised hyperintensity as seen in (E). Both findings are highly suggestive of a very small residual cholesteatoma pearl. Surgery revealed indeed a very small posteriorly and laterally located 3 mm small residual cholesteatoma pearl.

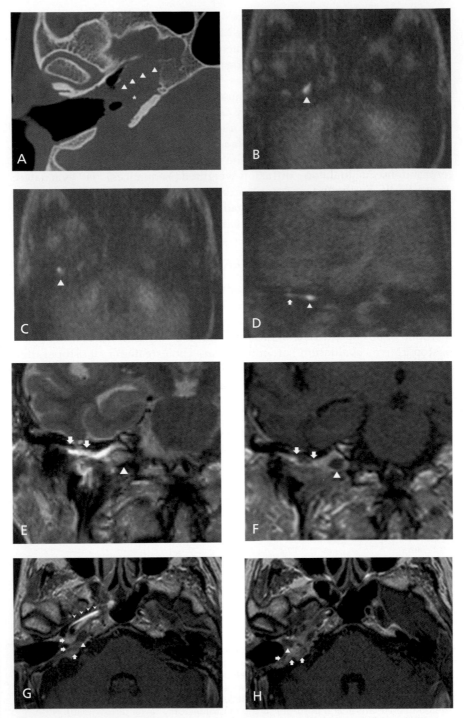

Fig. 7 A 65-year-old woman with extensive prior history of multiple cholesteatoma surgery finally resulting in a complete petrosectomy several years ago. The patient presented with right-sided pain situated in the petrosectomy cavity. This case demonstrates the superiority of non-echoplanar diffusion-weighted sequences in demonstrating post-operative recurrent cholesteatoma. Both cholesteatomas were confirmed on their suspected locations.

cholesteatoma. The rationale of this technique is based upon the fact that postoperative scar tissue and granulation tissue enhances slowly. Early scanning after intravenous gadolinium can cause false-positive findings. The main difference with the early reports on post-gadolinium T1-weighted imaging is that this protocol uses a delay of 45 min after i.v. gadolinium administration. By doing so, the postoperative scar and granulation tissue has the time to enhance, so differentiation with the non-enhancing cholesteatoma can be made. Using this protocol, residual cholesteatomas as small as 3 mm may be detected.

Major limitations, however, are the use of gadolinium which has become controversial due to the appearance of systemic fibrosis in patients with renal insufficiency. Furthermore, this protocol with unenhanced and late post-gadolinium T1-weighted enhanced images forms a time-consuming burden on the workflow of a radiology department.

Diffusion-weighted MR imaging

Echoplanar diffusion-weighted sequences were originally developed for the diagnosis of ischaemic brain lesions. This sequence is based upon the demonstration of movement of free water molecules and possible restriction of movement in the case of pathology.

Fig. 7 (continued)
(A) Axial CT image situated low in the petrosectomy cavity. The petrosectomy cavity is filled at its medial side by partially irregular dellneated soft tissues (asterisk). On CT, differentiation of these soft tissues is completely impossible. Note the loss of delineation of the intrapetrosal part of the carotid canal (arrowheads).
(B) Axial non-echoplanar diffusion-weighted image at the level of the skull base (right temporomandibular joint is just included in the slice). A nodular hyperintense lesion (arrowhead) can be seen on the right side just laterally to the moderately intense signal of the skull base. This nodular hyperintense lesion is highly suspicious for a small recurrent cholesteatoma.
(C) Axial non-echoplanar diffusion-weighted image, one slice higher than in (B). A second smaller nodular hyperintense lesion (arrowhead), already suspected in (B), situated laterally to the first lesion is seen. Again, this lesion is also highly suspicious of a second location of a recurrent cholesteatoma.
(D) Coronal non-echoplanar diffusion-weighted image at the level of the anterior skull base clearly shows the nodular lesion (arrowhead), located very medially in the skull base. The second very small lesion can already be suspected on this slice (arrow). This second very small lesion was better visualized on an adjacent slice (not shown).
(E) Coronal T2-weighted MR image (same level as [D]) shows the cholesteatoma as a nodular moderately intense lesion (arrowhead). The signal intensity of the cholesteatoma looks very similar to that of grey brain tissue in the adjacent temporal lobe. Note the intense signal of the associated scar and granulation tissue (arrows) situated laterally to the recurrent cholesteatoma.
(F) Coronal T1-weighted MR image (same level as in [D,E]) shows the cholesteatoma as a nodular non-enhancing lesion (arrowhead). Note the enhancing inflammatory and scar tissue lateral to the cholesteatoma partially filling up the resection cavity (arrows). The second smaller cholesteatoma can also be suspected as a small nodular non-enhancing lesion. Both lesions correspond to the visualized nodular hyperintensities on non-echoplanar diffusion-weighted sequences and are compatible with two recurrent cholesteatomas.
(G) Axial T1-weighted MR image (same level as in [A]). The cholesteatoma (large arrowhead) is embedded in enhancing scar tissue (arrows) with centrally non-enhancing cholesteatoma. Note that the cholesteatoma is in very close relationship to the intrapetrosal part of the internal carotid artery (small arrowheads).
(H) Axial T1-weighted MR image, one slice higher than (G). The second small cholesteatoma is seen as a small nodular hypo-intense lesion (arrowhead) embedded in enhancing scar and granulation tissue (arrows).

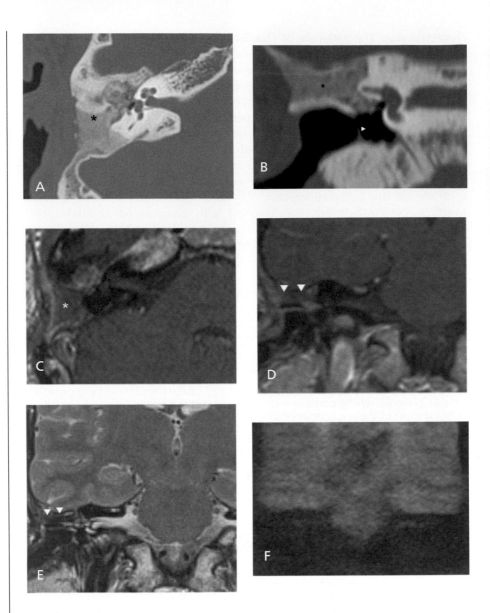

Fig. 8 A 27-year-old man with prior PBOT surgery for cholesteatoma. There is no evidence on CT or MRI for a residual or recurrent cholesteatoma.
(A) Axial CT image at the level of the internal auditory canal and the vestibule. The surgical cavity is completely filled up with a mixture of bone and bone paste (asterisk). Note the complete and homogeneous bone opacification of the cavity with bone. There are no punched-out lesions in the bony opacification.
(B) Coronal CT reconstructions at the level of the vestibule. Note, again, the complete opacification of the mastoidectomy cavity with bone (asterisk). There are no punched-out lesions in the bony filled up cavity. Note the well-aerated aspect of the middle ear (arrowhead).
(C) Axial late post-gadolinium T1-weighted image (same level as in [A]). Note the hypo-intense signal of the completely filled up cavity (asterisk). Signal intensities are aspecific but look somewhat like a cholesteatoma.
(D) Coronal late post-gadolinium T1-weighted image (same level as in [B]). Note, again, the somewhat inhomogeneous hypo-intense aspect of the filled cavity (arrowheads). It is difficult to exclude any cholesteatoma on this sequence.

Several reports have extensively described the use of echoplanar diffusion-weighted sequences in the diagnosis of middle-ear cholesteatoma.[13,14,26,27] Again, differentiation should be made between residual and recurrent cholesteatoma. According to Brackmann,[7] residual cholesteatoma is defined as cholesteatoma left behind at first-stage surgery whereas recurrent cholesteatoma usually starts as a new superoposterior retraction pocket. In our experience, residual cholesteatoma can be located anywhere in the middle ear and resection cavity and is much smaller than the recurrent cholesteatoma. This makes the detection of a residual cholesteatoma much more difficult. In a large series, we retrospectively reviewed the use of echoplanar diffusion-weighted sequence in the postoperative middle ear and mastoid cavities in order to evaluate its value to demonstrate these usually small residual cholesteatoma pearls.[14] Echoplanar diffusion-weighted imaging has (due to its limitations) a size limit of 5 mm in demonstrating middle-ear cholesteatoma. This makes echoplanar diffusion-weighted sequences useless for the detection of residual cholesteatomas. However, most reported studies using echoplanar diffusion-weighted sequences for the evaluation of postoperative cholesteatoma are studies on recurrent cholesteatomas.[26,27] All reported postoperative cholesteatomas are recurrent cholesteatomas and are much larger, being easily detectable using echoplanar diffusion-weighted sequences.[26]

It has already been reported that non-echoplanar based diffusion-weighted sequence have a higher sensitivity and specificity to detect cholesteatoma.[17] However, until now, only one report mentions the use of non-echoplanar based diffusion-weighted sequences for the evaluation of postoperative cholesteatoma.[18] Surprisingly, the reported cholesteatoma are again rather large recurrent cholesteatomas with a minimum size of 5 mm, equalling the detectable size of echoplanar diffusion-weighted sequences.[18]

Data from our own most recent results indicate that the non-echoplanar based diffusion-weighted sequences have a very high sensitivity and specificity in evaluating pre-second-look patients (Fig. 6).[28] Non-echoplanar diffusion-weighted imaging is able to detect very small residual cholesteatomas and has a high negative predictive and high positive predictive value. These results indicate that non-echoplanar diffusion-weighted sequences can select second look patients thus avoiding unnecessary interventions.[28] In our own data, the number of patients undergoing second-look surgery in our institution has dropped from about 65% to less than 10% using this technique.

In the case of a possible recurrent cholesteatoma, MRI is far superior to CT in the evaluation of these patients as CT usually only displays an aspecific soft tissue opacification of the resection cavity (Fig. 7). Further studies are currently in progress to evaluate whether one can start the evaluation of postoperative patients by using this non-echoplanar diffusion-weighted sequences alone.

Fig. 8 (*continued*)
(E) Coronal T2-weighted MR image (same level as in [B,D]). The signal of the obliterated cavity is homogeneous and very hypo-intense (arrowheads). Compare these to (C,D). Signal intensities on T1- and T2-weighted images are not at all compatible with cholesteatoma. The hypo-intense aspect on T1-weighted sequences and the very hypo-intense aspect on T2-weighted sequences are characteristic of an obliterated cavity.
(F) Coronal non-echoplanar diffusion-weighted image shows no hyperintensities at all. Recurrent or residual cholesteatoma can be excluded.

MRI OF PRIMARY BONY OBLITERATION TECHNIQUES

In primary bony obliteration techniques (PBOTs), a canal wall up procedure is used in combination with mainly bone and bone paté creating a bone density in the filled cavity. In these cases, a homogeneous aspect of the bony filled cavity should be noted (Fig. 8). Any punched-out soft tissue lesion into the obliterated and bony filled cavity is suspicious of a recurrent cholesteatoma.[10]

The signal intensities of such a filled cavity on standard MRI sequences are reported to be very inhomogeneous and mixed[10] making the diagnosis of a recurrent cholesteatoma impossible. A recent report on echoplanar diffusion-weighted images demonstrates the limitations of these sequences in the evaluation of the obliterated cavities as well as in the evaluation of an associated middle-ear cavity.[10]

Further studies are currently being undertaken to evaluate non-echoplanar based diffusion-weighted sequences in the evaluation of the PBOT as well as the associated (opacified) middle ear.

MRI PROTOCOL

Our current MRI protocol consists of the combination of both techniques and is mainly based on late post-gadolinium T1-weighted images and non-echoplanar diffusion-weighted sequences using a 1.5 T superconductive unit (Magnetom Avanto, Siemens Medical Solutions, Erlangen, Germany) with the standard Head Matrix coil. We no longer perform any unenhanced T1-weighted images. All sequences are performed 45 min after i.v. gadolinium administration.

Axial 2-mm thick spin-echo T1-weighted images (TR 400 ms, TE 17 ms, matrix 192 x 256, field of view 150 mm x 200 mm) and coronal 2-mm thick spin-echo T1-weighted images are acquired with the same parameters except for the matrix, which is set at 144 x 256 for the coronal images. Coronal 2-mm thick turbo spin-echo T2-weighted images (TR 3500 ms, TE 92 ms, matrix 192 x 256, field of view 150 mm x 200 mm) and axial 0.4-mm thick 3-D turbo spin-echo T2-weighted images (TR 1500 ms, TE 303 ms, matrix 228 x 448, field of view 107 mm x 210 mm) are also performed. In all patients, a 2-mm thick single-shot turbo spin-echo diffusion weighted sequence is acquired in the coronal plane (TR 2000 ms, TE 115 ms, matrix 134 x 192, field of view 220 mm x 220 mm, b factors 0 and 1000 mm^2/s). The coronal plane is preferred over the axial plane due to the fact that in the past, using EP-DW imaging, the coronal plane showed less artefacts. Out of habit, the coronal plane is still preferred.

CONCLUSIONS

For the evaluation of acquired and congenital cholesteatoma, MRI clearly has a complementary function to CT due to its superior soft tissue resolution and its ability to discriminate cholesteatoma from surrounding inflammation.

The combination of late post-gadolinium T1-weighted MR sequences and a non-echoplanar diffusion sequence has the highest sensitivity and specificity in the detection of postoperative residual or recurrent cholesteatoma. Therefore, evaluation of the postoperative middle ear should be done on MRI using the combination of both of these sequences.

Key points for clinical practice

- Cholesteatoma has an intermediate signal intensity on T2-weighted MR images, a hypo-intense signal with peripheral enhancement on T1-weighted images after i.v. gadolinium and a clear hyperintense signal on B1000 diffusion-weighted images.

- Non-echoplanar based diffusion-weighted sequences have the highest sensitivity and specificity for the detection of middle-ear cholesteatoma.

- Non-echoplanar based diffusion-weighted sequences are able to detect middle ear cholesteatoma as small as 2 mm whereas echo-planar diffusion-weighted sequences have a size limit of 5 mm.

- The evaluation of postoperative recurrent cholesteatoma has to be done on MRI using a protocol with late post-gadolinium T1-weighted and non-echo planar based diffusion-weighted rather than using CT.

- A state-of-the-art MRI protocol for cholesteatoma detection should include a combination of late (45 min) post-gadolinium T1-weighted sequence and a non-echoplanar based diffusion-weighted sequence.

References

1. Harnsberger R. *Diagnostic Imaging: Head and Neck*. Salt Lake City, UT: Amirsys, 2004.
2. Magluilo G. Petrous bone cholesteatoma: clinical longitudinal study. *Eur Arch Otorhinolaryngol* 2007; **264**: 115–120.
3. Nelson M, Roger G, Koltai PJ *et al*. Congenital cholesteatoma: classification, management and outcome. *Arch Otolaryngol Head Neck Surg* 2002; **128**: 810–814.
4. Lemmerling M, De Foer B. Imaging of cholesteatomatous and non-cholesteatomatous middle ear disease. In: Lemmerling M, Kollias S. (eds) *Radiology of the Petrous Bone*. Berlin: Springer, 2004; 31–47.
5. Shelton C, Sheehy JL. Tympanoplasty: review of 400 staged cases. *Laryngoscope* 1990; **100**: 679–681.
6. Darrouzet V, Duclos JY, Portmann D, Bebear JP. Preference for the closed technique in the management of cholesteatoma of the middle ear in children: a retrospective study of 215 consecutive patients treated over 10 years. *Am J Otol* 2000; **21**: 474–481.
7. Brackmann DE. Tympanoplasty with mastoidectomy: canal wall up procedures. *Am J Otol* 1993; **14**: 380–382.
8. Mercke U. The cholesteatomatous ear one year after surgery with obliteration technique. *Am J Otol* 1987; **8**: 534–536.
9. Gantz BJ, Wilkinson EP, Hansen MR. Canal wall reconstruction tympanomastoidectomy with mastoid obliteration. *Laryngoscope* 2005; **115**: 1734–1740.
10. De Foer B, Vercruysse JP, Pouilllon M *et al*. Value of high-resolution computed tomography and magnetic resonance imaging in the detection of residual cholesteatomas in primary bony obliterated mastoids. *Am J Otolaryngol* 2007; **28**: 230–234.
11. Lemmerling MM, De Foer B, Vandevyver V, Vercruysse JP, Verstraete KL. Imaging of the opacified middle ear. *Eur J Radiol* 2008; Mar 11 [Epub ahead of print]; PMID: 18339504 [PubMed - as supplied by publisher].
12. Martin N, Sterkers O, Nahum H. Chronic inflammatory disease of the middle ear cavities: Gd-DTPA-enhanced MR imaging. *Radiology* 1990; **176**: 399–405.
13. Fitzek C, Mewes T, Fitzek S *et al*. Diffusion-weighted MRI of cholesteatomas in petrous bone. *J Magn Reson Imaging* 2002; **15**: 636–641.
14. Vercruysse JP, De Foer B, Pouillon M *et al*. The value of diffusion-weighted MR imaging in the diagnosis of primary acquired and residual cholesteatoma: a surgical verified

study of 100 patients. *Eur Radiol* 2006; **16**: 1461–1467.

15. Huisman T. Diffusion-weighted imaging: basic concepts and application in cerebral stroke and head trauma. *Eur Radiol* 2003; **13**: 2283–2297.

16. Thoeny H, De Keyzer F. Extracranial applications of diffusion-weighted magnetic resonance imaging. *Eur Radiol* 2007; **17**: 1385–1393.

17. De Foer B, Vercruysse JP, Pilet B *et al.* Single-shot, turbo spin-echo, diffusion-weighted imaging versus spin-echo-planar, diffusion-weighted imaging in the detection of acquired middle ear cholesteatoma. *AJNR Am J Neuroradiol* 2006; **27**: 1480–1482.

18. Dubrulle F, Souillard R, Chechin D *et al.* Diffusion-weighted MR imaging sequence in the detection of postoperative recurrent cholesteatoma. *Radiology* 2006; **238**: 604–610.

19. De Foer B, Vercruysse JP, Bernaerts A *et al.* The value of single-shot turbo spin-echo diffusion-weighted MR imaging in the detection of middle ear cholesteatoma. *Neuroradiology* 2007; **49**: 841–848.

20. Robert Y, Carcasset S, Rocourt N *et al.* Congenital cholesteatoma of the temporal bone: MR findings and comparison with CT. *AJNR Am J Neuroradiol* 1995; **16**: 755–761.

21. Williams MT, Ayache D, Alberti C *et al.* Detection of post-operative residual cholesteatoma with delayed contrast-enhanced MR imaging: initial findings. *Eur Radiol* 2003; **13**: 169–174.

22. Ayache D, Williams MT, Lejeune D, Corré A. Usefulness of delayed postcontrast magnetic resonance imaging in the detection of residual cholesteatoma in the detection of residual cholesteatoma after canal wall-up tympanoplasty. *Laryngoscope* 2005; **115**: 607–610.

23. Tierney PA, Pracy P, Blaney SP, Bowdler DA. An assessment of the value of the preoperative computed tomography scans prior to otoendoscopic 'second look' in intact canal wall mastoid surgery. *Clin Otolaryngol Allied Sci* 1999; **24**: 274–276.

24. Blaney SP, Tierney P, Oyarazabal M, Bowdler DA. CT scanning in 'second look' combined approach tympanoplasty. *Rev Laryngol Otol Rhinol (Bord)* 2000; **121**: 79–81.

25. Wake M, Robinson JM, Witcombe JP *et al.* Detection of recurrent cholesteatoma by computerized tomography after 'closed cavity' mastoid surgery. *J Laryngol Otol* 1992; **106**: 393–395.

26. Aikele P, Kittner T, Offergeld C *et al.* Diffusion-weighted MR imaging of cholesteatoma in pediatric and adult patients who have undergone middle ear surgery. *AJR Am J Roentgenol* 2003; **181**: 261–265.

27. Stasolla A, Magluilo G, Parrotto D, Luppi G, Marini M. Detection of postoperative relapsing/residual cholesteatoma with diffusion-weighted echo-planar magnetic resonance imaging. *Otol Neurotol* 2004; **25**: 879–884.

28. De Foer B, Vercruysse J-P, Bernaerts A *et al.* Detection of postoperative residual cholesteatoma with non echo-planar diffusion-weighted magnetic resonance imaging. *Otol Neurotol* 2008; In press.

Richard A. Chole Osarenoma Olomu
Eric W. Wang

2

Bacterial biofilm infections in otology

Since van Leeuwenhoek first described single cell organisms in 1676,[1] most bacterial research has focused on individual free-swimming or planktonic organisms. However, most bacteria in nature exist in organized colonies termed biofilms. Bacterial biofilms are structured communities of sessile bacteria living in a secreted extracellular polymer matrix adherent to a surface.[2] The biofilm phenotype represents a distinct bacterial growth strategy, with unique gene and protein expression patterns. The biofilm phenotype provides a distinct survival advantage for the bacteria. Biofilms provide protection from environmental changes by creating a hydrated microniche that is less susceptible to the elements, more resistant to UV rays, osmotic stresses and fluctuations in the environment.[3] This survival advantage is further enhanced by complex intercellular signalling within the biofilm that alters the biofilm morphology as well as the gene expression of the bacteria within the matrix.[4,5] Bacterial biofilms are 3-dimensional structures with channels for nutrients, ions, water and waste. The biofilm matrix material can exclude materials or salvage materials to make the local environment more suitable to the bacteria.[3] The resulting differential gradient of nutrients and waste establishes microcolonies within the biofilm, providing additional microbial diversity and enhancing the survival of the biofilm. In nature, several

Richard A. Chole MD PhD (for correspondence)
Lindburg Professor and Chairman, Department of Otolaryngology, School of Medicine, Washington University in St Louis, Campus Box 8115, 660 South Euclid Ave, St Louis, MO 63110, USA
E-mail: rchole@wustl.edu

Osarenoma Olomu MD
Department of Otolaryngology, School of Medicine, Washington University in St Louis, Campus Box 8115, 660 South Euclid Ave, St Louis, MO 63110, USA

Eric W. Wang MD
Department of Otolaryngology, School of Medicine, Washington University in St Louis, Campus Box 8115, 660 South Euclid Ave, St Louis, MO 63110, USA

microbial species typically co-exist in a biofilm which may alter the structure of the biofilm and its ability to adapt to environmental stresses.

Importantly, biofilms are believed to contribute to a variety of chronic human diseases.[6] Most human pathogens can exist in biofilms. The ability of the bacteria to produce and maintain a biofilm is central to their ability to persist chronically in the body while evading natural host defences and antimicrobial therapy.[2] Microbial biofilms further exacerbate disease by providing a reservoir of bacteria that may now be resistant to antibiotics and are capable of seeding a new acute infection.[7] Examples of otological diseases that may be, at least partially, attributed to biofilms include chronic otitis media, cholesteatoma, and infection of middle ear devices such as middle ear prostheses and cochlear implants.

BIOFILM DEVELOPMENT

Biofilm formation is a well conserved, ancient phenotype.[8] There is evidence of bacteria growing in biofilms from samples of bacteria taken from 3000-year-old fossils. Biofilm formation is typically described in three stages: (i) attachment; (ii) growth of colonies; and (iii) detachment of planktonic organisms (Fig. 1). However, biofilm formation is a fluid process that is constantly adjusting to environmental changes. Intercellular communication occurs throughout biofilm formation and allows the community of microbes to respond to environmental stresses. When conditions allow for growth, the biofilm may respond by expanding through further attachment and production of extracellular matrix or changing the 3-dimensional structure. An overview of bacterial biofilm development provides a framework to understand biofilms and potential methods of inhibiting biofilm development.

ATTACHMENT

The first event in the formation of a biofilm is attachment of the bacteria to a surface. Bacteria are capable of attaching to surfaces in aqueous environments

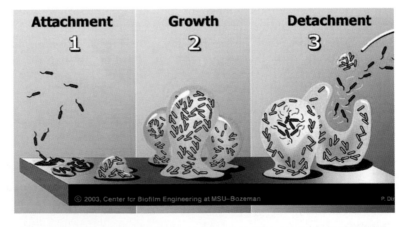

Fig. 1 Stages in biofilm development: (1) attachment; (2) growth of colonies; (3) detachment of planktonic organisms.

even in high-flow states. In industrial systems, bacteria have been shown to attach in Reynold's numbers exceeding 3000. Hence, biofilms can form on even the most fast-flowing fluid in the body, such as the heart valves. Upon attachment, the bacteria adhere irreversibly to the surface. This irreversible attachment is accompanied by a significant change in gene expression and results in a 'biofilm phenotype'.[2]

GROWTH OF COLONIES

The next stage is aggregation of the biofilm. The biofilm 'recruits' other bacteria as well as undergoing cell division within the colony. As the bacteria create a micro-environment within the biofilm, further changes in gene expression change the bacteria into a unique biofilm phenotype. In addition to intracellular changes, there is evidence of intercellular effects of biofilms. The bacteria within the biofilm 'communicate', are metabolically communal and enhance the survival of the colony, even at the expense of single cells. These intercellular networks have been especially studied in *Pseudomonas aeruginosa*.[4] At this stage of the colony's development, individual cells express quorum sensing genes in response to the environment. Quorum sensing is an intracellular signalling motif through which bacteria can communicate and co-ordinate gene expression by receiving and producing bacterial signalling molecules. Quorum sensing can initiate regulatory pathways and affect gene expression in multiple bacteria within the biofilm. It is primarily influenced by multiple environmental factors such as the surface the biofilm is attached to and the availability of various nutrients. It is one of the methods by which bacteria in biofilms can achieve division of labour, orient rapidly to a changing environment and, thus, ensure survival of some members of the colony.[5] Furthermore, it has been shown that some pathogenic strains of *P. aeruginosa* require quorum sensing to express certain virulence factors.[9]

Quorum sensing is also believed to initiate the production of extracellular matrix that provides the framework for the biofilm itself. The polymeric extracellular matrix is made up of a heterogeneous mixture of hydrated

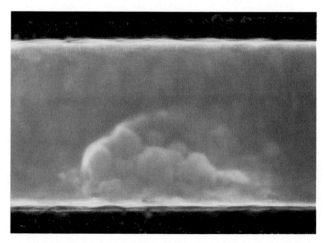

Fig. 2 *P. aeruginosa* biofilm in a 1-mm flow chamber seen under UV light. Live cells are green expressing green fluorescent protein.

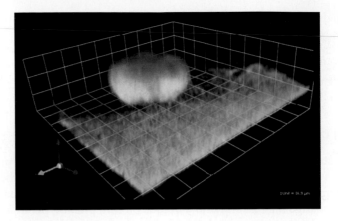

Fig. 3 A 3-dimensional confocal image of a mature *P. aeruginosa* biofilm. Live cells are green (expressing green fluorescent protein) and dead cells are red (live-dead stain).

polysaccharides including free DNA.[10] Also, in response to quorum sensing signals, the 3-dimensional structure of the biofilm develops, producing water channels distinct, micro-environments and nutrient gradients (Figs 2 and 3).

DETACHMENT AND RELEASE OF PLANKTONIC CELLS

The third stage of biofilm growth is detachment or dispersal of single bacterial cells or groups of cells (Fig. 1). This process can be active or passive, such as in shear stress. The process of separation is important to bacterial survival as it enhances the ability to colonize a new environment. In human disease, bacterial detachment from a biofilm may correspond to acute exacerbations of chronic infections.[6] The biofilm can serve as a nidus of the infection that survives attack by the host immune system and by antibiotics. As the biofilm sheds planktonic bacteria, infection may spread to distal sites as well as generate renewed symptoms. This is a postulated mechanism for recurrences of acute otitis media (OM) in individuals with chronic otitis media with effusion (OME).[11]

SURVIVAL MECHANISMS WITHIN BIOFILMS

Studies in natural environments and on industrial surfaces have shown enhanced survival of bacterial biofilm. In the last decade, research has shown how these enhanced survival mechanism assist pathogenesis in human diseases. The persistence of infection has been studied extensively in cystic fibrosis, where *P. aeruginosa* infection eventually colonizes the patient's lungs and develops into a biofilm that is virtually impossible to eradicate.[12] Established biofilms are highly resistant to host defences and antimicrobial agents. Whiteley *et al.*[13] showed that tobramycin-sensitive *P. aeruginosa* becomes highly resistant in its biofilm phenotype. Several mechanisms have been proposed to explain this resistance.[12] However, the aetiology of the antimicrobial resistance is likely multifactorial and may vary depending on the composition of the biofilm itself.

PHYSICAL BARRIERS

The structure of the biofilms provides a physical barrier which protects the colony from shear stress and changes in hydration and pH. Additionally the biofilm can become too large for phagocytosis.[7]

ANTIBIOTIC SEQUESTRATION AND DISRUPTION

Certain antibiotics may have limited or delayed diffusion through the biofilm matrix.[14–16]

ALTERED GROWTH RATE OR PERSISTER CELLS

Bacteria are more vulnerable to antibiotic therapy when multiplying rapidly. It has been shown that, at the core of several types of biofilms, there are slow-growing cells that often do not divide in a healthy biofilm. These slow-growing bacteria have been shown to be highly resistant to antibiotic therapy. It is proposed that they can survive the most aggressive antibiotic regimens and then act as a nidus for re-infection.[15,17]

EXCHANGE OF GENETIC MATERIAL

The exchange of genetic material in a dense biofilm colony is highly probable. *P. aeruginosa* is a well-studied biofilm organism and demonstrates significant genetic diversity. In addition to traditional methods of plasmid exchange, *P. aeruginosa* contains transposons within its genome that could facilitate the exchange of advantageous genetic material.[18]

RELEASE OR RESEEDING

The biofilm serves as a bacterial reserve that is capable of restarting an acute infection after therapy.[7]

NOVEL MECHANISMS

The intercellular interactions of bacteria within a biofilm is under intense investigation, but remains largely unknown at present. Novel mechanisms for evasion of host defence and antibiotics are possible.

BIOFILMS IN OTITIS MEDIA

Otitis media is the most common bacterial infection of childhood. It can be a chronic infection with effusion or a recurrent infection. Otitis media has significant economic and individual repercussions.[19] Two observations raised the possibility that OME and recurrent OM may be biofilm diseases. First, these processes seem to be chronic, indolent, inflammatory processes consistent with the presence of biofilms within the middle ear. Second, cultures of aspirated fluid are often sterile when bacterial DNA and RNA can be retrieved from the specimens.[20] Subsequently, Post *et al.*[11] showed evidence of biofilm

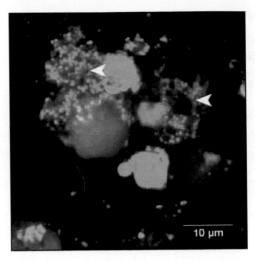

Fig. 4 Biofilms (arrowheads on an MEM specimen from an ear with an effusion that was PCR-positive for *Haemophilus influenzae*.[21]

formation in an animal model of otitis media. The most convincing evidence is from Hall-Stoodley *et al.*,[21] who detected anatomical evidence of bacterial biofilms on middle ear mucosa of children with OME and recurrent OM (see Fig. 4). The samples were obtained during tympanostomy tube placement and were detected by confocal microscopy, FISH, and PCR. Compared to controls, there is a biofilm presence on patients with OME and recurrent OM.

While the evidence that OME is a biofilm disease is strong, it is circumstantial. The presence of a biofilm on the mucosa of individuals with OME may be an epiphenomenon merely associated with the presence of an effusion in the middle ear. There is still evidence that at least some middle ear effusions show no evidence of bacterial genome.[22] It is clear that some middle ear effusions develop because of obstruction of the eustachian tube (hydrops *ex vacuo*) without biofilm formation. Dohar[23] pointed out that the failure of most cases of OME to persist argues against it being a biofilm disease. Confirmation that the aetiology of chronic OME or recurrent AOM is a microbial biofilm must wait until there are specific means to irradicate the biofilm selectively and the sessile bacteria within.

BIOFILMS IN INFECTED CHOLESTEATOMA

A defining feature of cholesteatoma is chronic and recurrent infections. An infected cholesteatoma develops chronic otorrhea that can be suppressed by antibiotic therapy. However, recurrence of infection with the same organism is common. It has been shown that mixed microbial biofilms grow in human cholesteatoma as well as in animal models of cholesteatoma.[24] As it is virtually impossible to clear these infections without complete removal of the cholesteatoma matrix, the recurrent nature of the diseases may be due to the persistence of antibiotic-resistant biofilms (Fig. 5).

A possible mechanism for the recurrent infection of cholesteatoma is survival of the bacteria within the biofilm matrix despite therapy. There is

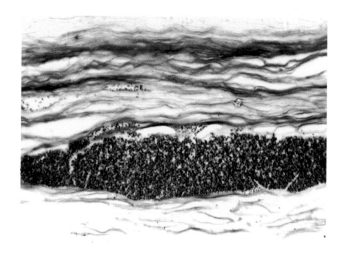

Fig. 5 A light micrograph of a mature biofilm within the keratin matrix of a human cholesteatoma. Toluidine blue, bacteria are dark staining.

evidence that *P. aeruginosa* associated with cholesteatoma from human samples are more capable of biofilm formation, with strong adherence to keratin-ocytes.[25] This evidence points to a potentially important role of biofilms in cholesteatoma formation and growth. Furthermore, the constant inflammation due to bacterial products from within the biofilm can play a role in the bony destruction seen in cholesteatoma. In our laboratory, we have shown how lipopolysaccharide (LPS) from *P. aeruginosa* can lead to osteoclastic bone resorption via the TLR4 receptor.[26] It is also possible that LPS and other products elaborated by a bacterial biofilm within the cholesteatoma matrix could lead to keratinocyte proliferation and, hence, rapid expansion of the cholesteatoma.

BIOFILMS AND MIDDLE EAR IMPLANT INFECTIONS

Bacterial biofilms have been detected in infected prostheses of many types including orthopaedic, urologic and cardiac implants.[27] Persistent inflammation and recurrent infection after the insertion of tympanostomy tube may be caused by persistent bacterial biofilms. Bothwell and colleagues[28] showed that a persistent *P. aeruginosa* infection resolved after the removal of a tympanostomy tube which had ultrastructural evidence of a bacterial biofilm.

The presence of biofilms on tympanostomy tubes is well established.[29] Cochlear implants removed because of persistent infection have also been shown to have anatomical evidence of biofilms.[30,31] The presence of bacterial biofilms on the surface of implants may explain the characteristic failure of these infections to be erradicated with appropriate antibiotics.

BIOFILMS IN CHRONIC OSTEORADIONECROSIS

Recently, we found evidence of biofilm formation in a case of osteoradionecrosis of the temporal bone.[32] Although the presence of a biofilm

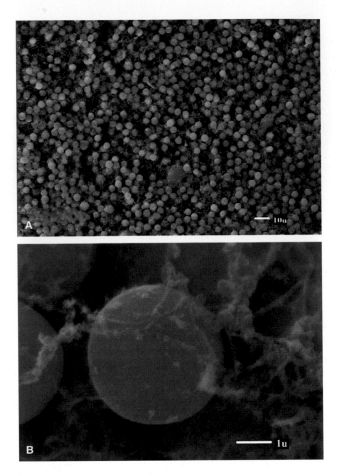

Fig. 6 (A) Low-power scanning electron micrograph of the peripheral part of the biofilm showing the matrix material is densely populated with *Staphylococcus aureus*. Bar = 10 μm. (B) High-power scanning electron micrograph image of the matrix material composed of EPS that are assumed to be from the host and the biofilm. This material has a complex structure that allows the bacteria to stay attached to a surface. Bar = 1 μm.[30]

on the surface of necrotic bone probably does not explain the pathogenesis of osteoradionecrosis, these bacteria may lead to persistence and progression of the bone destruction that is often seen with this disorder.

TREATMENT STRATEGIES FOR BACTERIAL BIOFILMS

Physical removal or disruption of a bacterial biofilm is effective in treating this chronic infection, but is often not clinically feasible. There are currently no specific, reliable alternative methods to prevent or irradicate microbial biofilms in patients. A number of strategies have been proposed and are under investigation. Jass and Lappin-Scott[33] found that low levels of electrical currents can enhance antibiotic efficacy against biofilms. Similarly, radio frequency alternating electric current (10 MHz) was shown to be effective in disrupting *Escherichia coli* biofilms.[34] Similarly, pulsed ultrasound may be an effective strategy in facilitating the transport of antibiotics throughout a mature biofilm.[35]

Furanones, found in red algae, have been shown to inhibit biofilm formation by inhibiting a key bacterial quorum-sensing pathway, the acylated homoserine lactone regulatory system in Gram-negative bacteria.[36,37]

Studies have shown that some macrolide antibiotics (*i.e.* clarithromycin and erythromycin) may be effective in killing sessile bacteria within biofilms.[38] Furthermore, some macrolides inhibit biofilm formation, possibly because of properties other than bactericidal activity.[39] In patients with chronic pulmonary inflammatory syndromes, macrolides show immunomodulatory effects.

We have shown that gentian violet and ferric ammonium citrate inhibit *P. aeruginosa* biofilms *in vitro*.[40] In a screen of 4509 compounds, Musk and colleagues[41] found that iron salts effectively inhibited biofilm formation in *Pseudomonas* spp. They concluded that iron inhibits the expression of certain genes essential for biofilm production. Since these iron salts are well tolerated biologically and inhibit biofilms of *Pseudomonas* spp. at low concentrations, they may be an efficient way of treating biofilm diseases *in vivo*.

CONCLUSIONS

Evidence supports the role of bacterial biofilms in several chronic otological infections including chronic otitis media, cholesteatoma and otological prostheses. The hallmark of bacterial biofilms is the increased resistance to antibiotics and host defences. The mechanisms for this resistance are under investigation. Similarly, novel mechanisms and alternatives to traditional antibiotics for the inhibition and eradication of biofilms is an area of active study.

Key points for clinical practice

- Chronic biofilm infections are common on otolaryngologic diseases

- Chronic biofilm infections are highly resistant to antibiotics and host defenses

- Eradication of biofilm infections usually requires removal.

References

1. Porter JR. Antony van Leeuwenhoek: tercentenary of his discovery of bacteria. *Bacteriol Rev* 1976; **40**: 260–269.
2. Costerton JW, Stewart PS, Greenberg EP. Bacterial biofilms: a common cause of persistent infections. *Science* 1999; **284**: 1318–1322.
3. Costerton JW, Lewandowski Z, DeBeer D, Caldwell D, Korber D, James G. Biofilms, the customized microniche. *J Bacteriol* 1994; **176**: 2137–2142.
4. Kirisits MJ, Parsek MR. Does *Pseudomonas aeruginosa* use intercellular signalling to build biofilm communities? *Cell Microbiol* 2006; **8**: 1841–1849.
5. Davies DG, Parsek MR, Pearson JP, Iglewski BH, Costerton JW, Greenberg EP. The involvement of cell-to-cell signals in the development of a bacterial biofilm. *Science* 1998; **280**: 295–298.

6. Potera C. Forging a link between biofilms and disease. *Science* 1999; **283**: 1837–1839.
7. Stewart PS, Costerton JW. Antibiotic resistance of bacteria in biofilms. *Lancet* 2001; **358**: 135–138.
8. Reysenbach AL, Cady SL. Microbiology of ancient and modern hydrothermal systems. *Trends Microbiol* 2001; **9**: 79–86.
9. Hentzer M, Wu H, Andersen JB *et al.* Attenuation of *Pseudomonas aeruginosa* virulence by quorum sensing inhibitors. *EMBO J* 2003; **22**: 3803–3815.
10. Whitchurch CB, Tolker-Nielsen T, Ragas PC, Mattick JS. Extracellular DNA required for bacterial biofilm formation. *Science* 2002; **295**: 1487.
11. Post JC. Direct evidence of bacterial biofilms in otitis media. *Laryngoscope* 2001; **111**: 2083–2094.
12. Coquet L, Junter GA, Jouenne T. Resistance of artificial biofilms of *Pseudomonas aeruginosa* to imipenem and tobramycin. *J Antimicrob Chemother* 1998; **42**: 755–760.
13. Whiteley M, Bangera MG, Bumgarner RE *et al.* Gene expression in *Pseudomonas aeruginosa* biofilms. *Nature* 2001; **413**: 860–864.
14. Anderl JN, Franklin MJ, Stewart PS. Role of antibiotic penetration limitation in *Klebsiella pneumoniae* biofilm resistance to ampicillin and ciprofloxacin. *Antimicrob Agents Chemother* 2000; **44**: 1818–1824.
15. Walters 3rd MC, Roe F, Bugnicourt A, Franklin MJ, Stewart PS. Contributions of antibiotic penetration, oxygen limitation, and low metabolic activity to tolerance of *Pseudomonas aeruginosa* biofilms to ciprofloxacin and tobramycin. *Antimicrob Agents Chemother* 2003; **47**: 317–323.
16. Brooun A, Liu S, Lewis K. A dose-response study of antibiotic resistance in *Pseudomonas aeruginosa* biofilms. *Antimicrob Agents Chemother* 2000; **44**: 640–646.
17. Lewis K. Persister cells and the riddle of biofilm survival. *Biochemistry (Mosc)* 2005; **70**: 267–274.
18. Mah TF, Pitts B, Pellock B, Walker GC, Stewart PS, O'Toole GA. A genetic basis for *Pseudomonas aeruginosa* biofilm antibiotic resistance. *Nature* 2003; **426**: 306–310.
19. Bennett KE, Haggard MP, Silva PA, Stewart IA. Behaviour and developmental effects of otitis media with effusion into the teens. *Arch Dis Child* 2001; **85**: 91–95.
20. Rayner MG, Zhang Y, Gorry MC, Chen Y, Post JC, Ehrlich GD. Evidence of bacterial metabolic activity in culture-negative otitis media with effusion. *JAMA* 1998; **279**: 296–299.
21. Hall-Stoodley L, Hu FZ, Gieseke A *et al.* Direct detection of bacterial biofilms on the middle-ear mucosa of children with chronic otitis media. *JAMA* 2006; **296**: 202–211.
22. Fergie N, Bayston R, Pearson JP, Birchall JP. Is otitis media with effusion a biofilm infection? *Clin Otolaryngol Allied Sci* 2004; **29**: 38–46.
23. Dohar J. Evidence that otitis media is not a biofilm disease. *Ear Nose Throat J* 2007; **86**: 1–12.
24. Chole RA, Faddis BT. Evidence for microbial biofilms in cholesteatomas. *Arch Otolaryngol Head Neck Surg* 2002; **128**: 1129–1133.
25. Wang EW, Jung JY, Pashia ME, Nason R, Scholnick S, Chole RA. Otopathogenic *Pseudomonas aeruginosa* strains as competent biofilm formers. *Arch Otolaryngol Head Neck Surg* 2005; **131**: 983–989.
26. Zhuang L, Jung JY, Wang EW *et al. Pseudomonas aeruginosa* lipopolysaccharide induces osteoclastogenesis through a Toll-like receptor 4 mediated pathway *in vitro* and *in vivo*. *Laryngoscope* 2007; **117**: 841–847.
27. Costerton JW, Montanaro L, Arciola CR. Biofilm in implant infections: its production and regulation. *Int J Artif Organs* 2005; **28**: 1062–1068.
28. Bothwell MR, Smith AL, Phillips T. Recalcitrant otorrhea due to *Pseudomonas* biofilm. *Otolaryngol Head Neck Surg* 2003; **129**: 599–601.
29. Jang CH, Cho YB, Choi CH. Structural features of tympanostomy tube biofilm formation in ciprofloxacin-resistant *Pseudomonas* otorrhea. *Int J Pediatr Otorhinolaryngol* 2007; **71**: 591–595.
30. Pawlowski KS, Wawro D, Roland PS. Bacterial biofilm formation on a human cochlear implant. *Otol Neurotol* 2005; **26**: 972–975.
31. Antonelli PJ, Lee JC, Burne RA. Bacterial biofilms may contribute to persistent cochlear implant infection. *Otol Neurotol* 2004; **25**: 953–957.

32. Nason R, Chole RA. Bacterial biofilms may explain chronicity in osteoradionecrosis of the temporal bone. *Otol Neurotol* 2007; **28**: 1026–1028.
33. Jass J, Lappin-Scott HM. The efficacy of antibiotics enhanced by electrical currents against *Pseudomonas aeruginosa* biofilms. *J Antimicrob Chemother* 1996; **38**: 987–1000.
34. Caubet R, Pedarros-Caubet F, Chu M *et al*. A radio frequency electric current enhances antibiotic efficacy against bacterial biofilms. *Antimicrob Agents Chemother* 2004; **48**: 4662–4664.
35. Carmen JC, Nelson JL, Beckstead BL *et al*. Ultrasonic-enhanced gentamicin transport through colony biofilms of *Pseudomonas aeruginosa* and *Escherichia coli*. *J Infect Chemother* 2004; **10**: 193–199.
36. de Nys R, Givskov M, Kumar N, Kjelleberg S, Steinberg PD. Furanones. *Prog Mol Subcell Biol* 2006; **42**: 55–86.
37. Manefield M, de Nys R, Kumar N *et al*. Evidence that halogenated furanones from *Delisea pulchra* inhibit acylated homoserine lactone (AHL)-mediated gene expression by displacing the AHL signal from its receptor protein. *Microbiology* 1999; **145**: 283–291.
38. Yasuda H, Ajiki Y, Koga T, Yokota T. Interaction between clarithromycin and biofilms formed by *Staphylococcus epidermidis*. *Antimicrob Agents Chemother* 1994; **38**: 138–141.
39. Amsden GW. Anti-inflammatory effects of macrolides – an underappreciated benefit in the treatment of community-acquired respiratory tract infections and chronic inflammatory pulmonary conditions? *J Antimicrob Chemother* 2005; **55**: 10–21.
40. Wang EW, Olumu O, Agostini G, Chole RA. *Pseudomonas aeruginosa* biofilms in flow chambers are inhibited by gentian violet and ferrous ammonium citrate. Abstract of the Triological Society, 2007.
41. Musk DJ, Banko DA, Hergenrother PJ. Iron salts perturb biofilm formation and disrupt existing biofilms of *Pseudomonas aeruginosa*. *Chem Biol* 2005; **12**: 789–796.

Thomas Lenarz Hubert H. Lim Minoo Lenarz

3

Auditory midbrain implant: experimental and clinical results

Deep brain stimulation for hearing restoration in patients with neural deafness has become more widely accepted since 1979, when a simple bipolar ball electrode was implanted on the surface of the cochlear nucleus.[1] Over the past 30 years, the cochlear nucleus has remained the main target for central auditory prostheses. The auditory brainstem implant (ABI) was first, and is still mostly, used in neurofibromatosis type 2 (NF2) patients whose auditory nerves were destroyed either by, or during, resection of VIIIth nerve tumours (Fig. 1). The fact that the cochlear nucleus is approached during tumour removal has justified its selection as a site for an auditory prosthesis. The current ABI system is similar to that of the cochlear implant, in which the only major difference is in the form of the micro-electrode array (Fig. 2). Currently, more than 500 NF2 patients world-wide are implanted with the ABI, which provides these subjects with improvements in environmental awareness and lip-reading capabilities. Unfortunately, only a small percentage of NF2 recipients achieve some open set speech perception without lip-reading. The overall performance in NF2 patients is not comparable, therefore, to the present multichannel cochlear implants, which can restore open set speech understanding without lip reading in postlingually deafened adults and even enable patients to converse over the telephone.[2-4]

Thomas Lenarz MD PhD
Professor and Director of the Otolaryngology Department, Medical University of Hannover, Carl-Neubergstr. 1, 30625 Hannover, Germany. Tel: +49 (0)511/532-6565
E-mail: ric@hno.mh-hannover.de; lenarz.thomas@mh-hannover.de

Hubert H. Lim PhD
Postdoctoral Research Scientist, Otolaryngology Department, Medical University of Hannover, Carl-Neubergstr. 1, 30625 Hannover, Germany. E-mail: hubertlim@aol.com

Minoo Lenarz MD (for correspondence)
Otolaryngologist and Neck Surgeon, Assistant Professor in the Otolaryngology Department, Medical University of Hannover, Carl-Neubergstr. 1, 30625 Hannover, Germany.
E-mail: Lenarz.Minoo@MH-Hannover.de

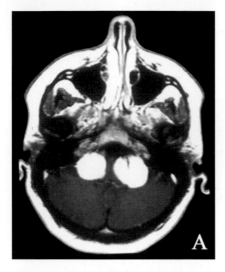
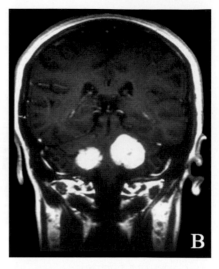

Fig. 1 The T1-weighted magnetic resonance imaging in axial (A) and coronal (B) views showing the bilateral acoustic neuromas in an NF2 patient (white circular areas). Large acoustic neuromas with brainstem compression and displacement are frequently observed in NF2 patients. This compression as well as the surgical trauma during tumour removal may cause damage to the cochlear nucleus and result in limited hearing performance with auditory brainstem implants in NF2 patients.

Recently, ABI implementation has been extended to another category of candidates who also can not benefit from cochlear implants (*e.g.* those with post-traumatic cochlear nerve avulsion or inaccessible cochleae due to severe ossification resulting from meningitis or otosclerosis). In contrast to the NF2 ABI patients, some of these non-tumour recipients perform significantly better and are capable of understanding speech without lip-reading. The fact that the same surface ABI technology in a similar location produces far better results in some of these non-tumour patients supports the hypothesis that tumour-induced damage in the cochlear nucleus may be responsible for the limited success of ABI in NF2 patients.[5]

Therefore, an alternative implantation site that bypasses the damaged pathways in the brainstem may provide better hearing performance in NF2 patients. This was the rationale for developing a new central auditory prosthesis for penetrating stimulation of the inferior colliculus (IC), particularly its central nucleus (ICC), in the auditory midbrain (Figs 2–4).

THE INFERIOR COLLICULUS

The IC is an anatomically well-defined and surgically accessible structure in the human auditory midbrain.[6–9] The human IC has a diameter of about 6–7 mm in all planes of section. It is located at the dorsal surface of the midbrain and is an obligatory synaptic terminus for almost all ascending auditory pathways.[10] The main projection area of the ascending input is the ICC, in which virtually every kind of preprocessed auditory information from the brainstem is collected.

One of the main reasons for selecting the ICC as a site for an auditory implant, in addition to providing access to almost all ascending auditory

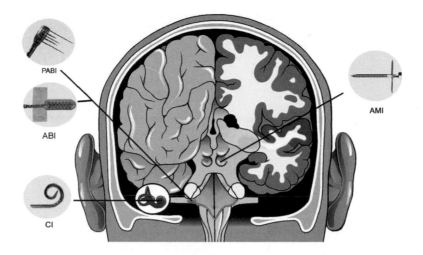

Fig. 2 Simplified schematic of the brain depicting the locations of the different auditory prosthetic arrays currently implanted into humans. Both the PABI and AMI are in clinical trials. All the shown devices have been developed by Cochlear Ltd (Lane Cove, Australia) though other ABIs and CIs have been developed by various companies. CI, cochlear implant; ABI, auditory brainstem implant; PABI, penetrating auditory brainstem implant; AMI, auditory midbrain implant. Taken from Lenarz *et al.*[13] and reprinted with permission from Lippincott Williams & Wilkins.

information, is its well-defined tonotopic organisation,[9] which appears to be important for an auditory prosthesis.[11] The ICC is different from the other subdivisions of the IC (*i.e.* dorsomedial nucleus, dorsal cortex, lateral zone) with its laminated neuropil composed mostly of disc-shaped neurons with their long axes aligned in parallel so as to form dendritic layers. Such layers establish a striated pattern in sections through the ICC that are parallel to the incoming layers of the lateral lemniscus. These morphological features are relatively consistent in the mammalian phylogeny and embryogenesis. Detailed studies with Golgi-impregnated sections and other staining methods have shown that this layered organisation in animals is similar in almost every respect to that of the human.[7–9] Animal studies have demonstrated a strong correlation between the laminar arrangement of neurons and the tonotopic organisation of the ICC.[9] For example, the planes of orientation of cellular laminae in cat ICC approximately align with the frequency-band laminae. In cat, there appears to be about 35–40 of these frequency-band laminae (each 175 ± 83 μm wide) where the lowest frequencies are represented dorsolaterally and the higher frequencies are represented more ventromedially.[12] In humans, it has also been shown that the ICC consists of layers that are analogous to those observed in other species (Fig. 3).[7] As has been demonstrated across different species, these layers should correspond to different frequency laminae.

Based on anatomical results presented by Geniec and Morest,[7] the human ICC is roughly 3.5 mm along its tonotopic dimension. It is not clear how thick the individual ICC laminae are since there do not appear to be any obvious boundaries between the layers. However, based on the similarities between human and cat with respect to the anatomical structure of the ICC and

35

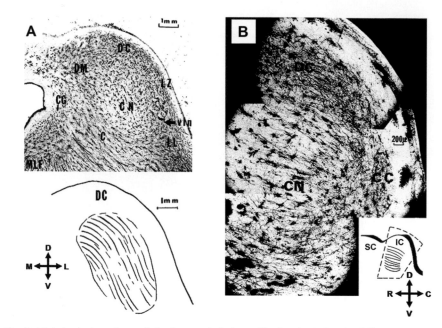

Fig. 3 Histological sections of the human inferior colliculus depicting its different subdivisions and layered structure using the Golgi–Cox method (taken from Geniec and Morest[7] and reprinted with permission from Taylor and Francis Group). (A) Axial section (top) at the junction of the caudal and middle thirds of the inferior colliculus of a 55-year-old man, and its simplified schematic (bottom) showing the orientation of the dendritic laminae within the central nucleus. (B) Parasagittal section at the junction of the medial and middle thirds of the inferior colliculus of a 53-year-old man; inset provides orientation of the dendritic laminae within the central nucleus and indicates the location of the section (dashed lines). C, cuneiform area; CC, caudal cortex; CG, central grey; CN, central nucleus; DC, dorsal cortex; DM, dorsomedial nucleus; IC, inferior colliculus; LL, lateral nucleus and dorsal nucleus of lateral lemniscus; LZ, lateral zone; MLF, medial longitudinal fasciculus; SC, superior colliculus; vln, ventrolateral nucleus.

thicknesses of the disc-shaped neurons making up the laminae,[7–9,12] it is likely that the frequency laminae in humans will span roughly 200 μm in thickness.

AUDITORY MIDBRAIN IMPLANT

The auditory midbrain implant (AMI; Cochlear Ltd, Lane Cove, Australia) is a single-shank multi-electrode array designed according to the dimensions of the human IC with the goal of stimulating the different layers of the ICC (Fig. 4).[13] The AMI electrode array is 6.4 mm long, with a diameter of 0.4 mm. It consists of 20 platinum ring electrodes linearly spaced at an interval of 200 μm. Each site has a width of 100 μm (surface area of 126,000 μm^2) and is connected to a parylene-coated, 25-μm thick wire (90% platinum/10% iridium). The body (carrier) of the electrode array is made from silicone rubber (30 durometer hardness) and is concentrically hollow. A stiffening element (stylet) made of stainless steel is positioned through the axial centre of this silicone carrier to enable insertion of the electrode array into the IC. After the electrode array is in its final position, the stylet will be removed, and the softer silicone carrier will remain in the tissue. A Dacron mesh is used to anchor the electrode array

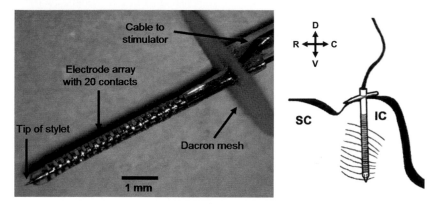

Fig. 4 Image of the AMI array with a schematic (right) depicting the orientation of the array along the tonotopic layers of the central nucleus of the IC. IC, inferior colliculus; SC, superior colliculus. Taken from Lenarz et al.[13] and reprinted with permission from Lippincott Williams & Wilkins.

onto the surface of the neural tissue to minimise movement after implantation. This Dacron mesh also prevents over insertion of the electrode array into the IC during implantation.

The other components of the AMI system are similar to the latest Nucleus cochlear implant system (Cochlear Ltd) consisting of a behind-the-ear microphone and processor that transmits the electromagnetic signals to the receiver-stimulator implanted under the skin. This receiver-stimulator is implanted in a bony bed on the skull near the craniotomy and is connected with a cable to the electrode array.

ELECTROPHYSIOLOGICAL FEASIBILITY

One major rationale for selecting the ICC as the target site for an auditory prosthesis is its well-defined tonotopic organisation. We designed our AMI array based on this organisation and the dimensions of the human IC, and hypothesised that AMI stimulation of the ICC would achieve frequency-specific activation. Furthermore, we expected lower thresholds than cochlear implant stimulation because of the ability to stimulate ICC neurons directly compared to the distant nature of neural activation (across the bony modiolar wall) for cochlear stimulation. The AMI sites are large due to limitations in electrode development technology. Yet this should also result in lower charge densities for ICC activation, thus providing a safer range of current levels for central nervous system stimulation.

To test our hypotheses, we performed experiments in a ketamine-anaesthetised guinea pig model in which we electrically stimulated different regions along the tonotopic axis of the ICC and recorded the corresponding neural activity across the tonotopic gradient of the primary auditory cortex (A1; Fig. 5). We used single biphasic monopolar pulses (200 µs/phase, cathodic-leading) within the ICC where the return was through a wire positioned in a neck muscle. Each ICC site was stimulated with levels between 1–100 µA in logarithmic (dB) steps for 40 trials, including 40 no-stimulus

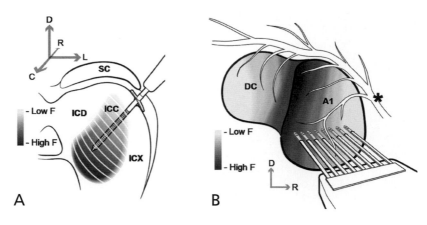

Fig. 5 Drawings of the AMI array and an 8-shank silicon-substrate Michigan probe (Center for Neural Communication Technology, University of Michigan, Ann Arbor, MI, USA) positioned along the tonotopic gradient of ICC (A) and A1 (B), respectively. Anatomy in (A) and (B) was derived from images presented in Malmierca et al.[44] and Wallace et al.,[45] respectively (not drawn to scale). Electrode sites (~400 μm²) are represented by black dots along each A1 probe shank (sites separated by 50 μm, shanks separated by 200 μm). The asterisk corresponds to blood vessels. A1, primary auditory cortex; DC, dorsocaudal cortex; F, frequency; ICC, inferior colliculus central nucleus; ICD, inferior colliculus dorsal cortex; ICX, inferior colliculus external cortex; SC, superior colliculus. Taken from Lenarz et al.[14] and reprinted with permission from Springer.

(spontaneous) trials, all in a randomised sequence at two presentations per second. The A1 neural activity (evoked potentials and spikes) was filtered and processed for analysis. Further details are presented in Lenarz et al.[14]

Figure 6 presents ICC stimulation thresholds for A1 spike activation. The mean value for the BF-aligned thresholds was 27.4 μA (SD 12.3 μA) and the mean value for the lowest-aligned thresholds was 20.7 μA (SD 9.6 μA). For cochlear stimulation, A1 thresholds of about 67.2 μA (median value) have been reported,[15] which is 10 dB higher than our median value of 20 μA. Even accounting for differences in the threshold method used, these results suggest that the AMI may provide lower thresholds than cochlear implants, which could potentially reduce overall energy consumption during daily use. Furthermore, current levels for AMI activation should be safe for central nervous system stimulation. Our thresholds ranged from about 6–60 μA, which for a 200 μs/phase pulse results in a total charge per phase of 1.2–12 nC. For 126,000 μm² sites, this results in a charge density per phase ranging between about 1–10 μC/cm². Using a charge density per phase of about 10 μC/cm² (7 h of continuous stimulation at 50 Hz, anodic-leading biphasic pulses, 400 μs/phase) in cat parietal cortex, McCreery et al.[16] demonstrated that safe neural stimulation up to 5000 nC/phase was possible. Even with differences in stimulation parameters and brain region, this charge per phase value is substantially higher than what was observed for our AMI thresholds (< 12 nC/phase). We could not determine the maximum current level needed for AMI stimulation with our experimental set-up. However, even if levels reach up to 500 μA, the total charge per phase and charge density per phase will still only be about 100 nC and 80 μC/cm², respectively, which is still well within the safe limits presented elsewhere.[16,17] In the next section, we further

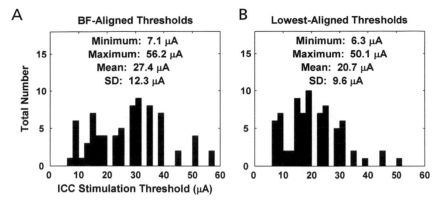

Fig. 6 (A) Electrical thresholds for neural activation on A1 sites with the closest BF to the stimulated AMI sites (*n* = 75). (B) Electrical thresholds for neural activation on A1 sites (selected from all 16 sites for a given A1 probe placement) with the lowest threshold for the stimulated AMI sites (*n* = 75). Taken from Lenarz *et al*.[14] and reprinted with permission from Springer.

demonstrate that current levels within the operating range of hearing do not induce any additional tissue damage above what is caused by the implanted AMI array.

To assess frequency-specificity of ICC stimulation, we plotted the BF of the A1 site that elicited the lowest threshold of activation for stimulation of a given ICC site against the BF of that stimulated ICC site (Fig. 7A). It was not always the case that stimulation of a given ICC site elicited the lowest threshold on the A1 site with the closest BF to the stimulated site. In several cases, the lowest

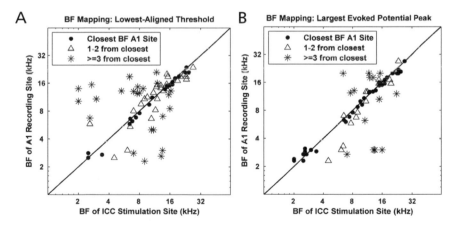

Fig. 7 BF mapping plots demonstrating that ICC stimulation with our AMI array achieves frequency-specific activation. (A) The BF of the A1 site with the lowest threshold for a stimulated AMI site is plotted against the BF of that AMI site. Diagonal line depicts perfect mapping, which is not always possible due to the set geometry of the electrode sites thus inherent BF misalignment. Symbols: ·, closest BF site; Δ, 1–2 sites away from closest BF site; *, > 2 sites away. Distribution of symbols: ·, *n* = 23; Δ, *n* = 27; *, *n* = 25. (B) The BF of the A1 site with the largest evoked potential peak for a stimulated AMI site (at 5 dB above threshold) is plotted against the BF of that AMI site. Symbols: ·, closest BF site; Δ, 1–2 sites away from closest BF site; *, > 2 sites away. Distribution of symbols: ·, *n* = 37; Δ, *n* = 16; *, *n* = 16. Taken from Lenarz *et al*.[14] and reprinted with permission from Springer.

threshold site could have a BF several sites away from that of the stimulated site. However, ICC stimulation generally achieved frequency-specific activation, in which 67% of the stimulated sites were less than or equal to two sites away from the closest BF site (*i.e.* neighbouring sites 200 μm away). What is also important is whether or not frequency-specific activation is maintained for higher levels, which corresponds more to the operating range for daily hearing. To obtain a global measure of activation across multiple A1 neurons, we measured the negative peak magnitude of the evoked potential recorded on each A1 site in response to stimulation of each ICC site. We then plotted the BF of the A1 site with the largest magnitude for stimulation of a given ICC site against the BF of the stimulated site (Fig. 7B) at a level 5 dB above spike threshold. A total of 77% of the stimulated ICC sites elicited the largest evoked potential on an A1 site with a similar BF (≤2 sites away). These results demonstrate that frequency-specific activation is achievable within the ICC using our AMI array at threshold and higher levels. However, there were some cases where this frequency-specificity was degraded, which may reflect effects of location of stimulation within the ICC and recording within A1.

Our electrophysiological findings are consistent with those presented by Lim and Anderson.[18,19] Furthermore, those studies suggest that location of stimulation within the ICC can affect different coding features, such as those associated with thresholds, evoked potential magnitudes, latencies, temporal features, level discrimination steps, and even spectral processing. Therefore, it is important to determine if similar stimulation location effects occur in humans and to identify the appropriate regions for ICC implantation and activation to restore useful hearing.

HISTOMORPHOLOGICAL EFFECTS

In order to pursue clinical trials, we needed to demonstrate that the AMI not only has potential as an auditory prosthesis but also is safe for chronic implantation and stimulation of the IC. To investigate its safety for clinical use, we assessed the histomorphological effects of chronic implantation and stimulation of the array within the feline IC, which is similar in cyto-architecture and size to the human IC. Eight cats were chronically implanted for 3 months; four of these were additionally stimulated for 60 days (4 h/day) starting 4 weeks after implantation to assess if clinically relevant stimuli further affected the tissue response. The stimuli consisted of cathodic-leading, charge-balanced pulses in common ground mode (100 μs/phase, 250 pps, 45 μs phase gap) using the SPEAK strategy (Cochlear Ltd) and driven by continuous sound from a radio. Across animals and throughout the 3-month implant period, the threshold (T) and comfortable (C) levels used to programme the processor ranged from 84–209 μA and 93–256 μA, respectively. A more detailed description of the methods and analyses are presented in Lenarz *et al.*[20]

In our experiments, we analysed the histomorphological effects 3 months after initial array implantation, which generally corresponds to the long-term sustained tissue response. In Giemsa-stained sections, the electrode tracks in both non-stimulated and stimulated cats were surrounded by a thin fibrillary sheath (Figs 8 and 9). There was no significant difference in the thickness of the reactive fibrillary sheath between the non-stimulated and stimulated cats

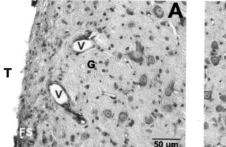
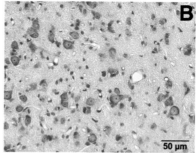

Fig. 8 Giemsa-stained histological sections showing the distribution of neurons and glial cells adjacent to the track of a chronically implanted non-stimulated electrode array (A) in comparison to those in a similar location in the contralateral (control) IC of the same cat (B). The fibrillary sheath around the track can also be seen. FS, fibrillary sheath; G, glial cell; N, neuron; T, track; V, vessel. Taken from Lenarz et al.[20] and reprinted with permission from Lippincott Williams & Wilkins.

suggesting that the encapsulation process is more affected by the implantation of a foreign object rather than chronic stimulation. The average thickness of the fibrillary sheath across all non-stimulated and stimulated data was 58.1 µm (SD 62.7 µm). Around the fibrillary sheath, reactive gliosis was detected in both non-stimulated and stimulated cats (Figs 8 and 9). The stimulated cats exhibited significant elevation of glial cells out to about 250 µm from the electrode track, while the non-stimulated cats had elevated glial cells out to about 350 µm (Fig. 10C,D). Intact and healthy neurons could be observed around the electrode track in both stimulated and non-stimulated ICs (Figs 8 and 9). However, there were fewer neurons in the immediate vicinity of the electrode tracks in both animal groups. The neuron density increased to normal at about 50 µm from the track in the stimulated cats and at about 100 µm from the track in non-stimulated cats (Fig. 10A,B). In comparing the plots in Figure 10, it is apparent that the extent of neuronal survival is inversely related to the level of glial reaction such that a greater number of glial cells corresponds to a fewer number of neurons at each distance from the electrode

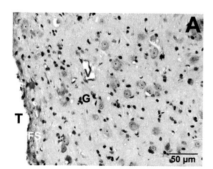
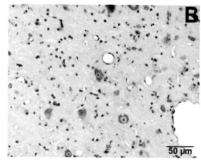

Fig. 9 Giemsa-stained histological sections showing the distribution of neurons and glial cells adjacent to the track of a chronically stimulated electrode array (A) in comparison to those in a similar location in the contralateral (control) IC of the same cat (B). The fibrillary sheath around the track can also be seen. FS, fibrillary sheath; G, glial cell; N, neuron; T, track; V, vessel. Taken from Lenarz et al.[20] and reprinted with permission from Lippincott Williams & Wilkins.

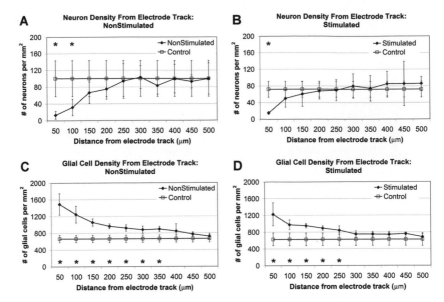

Fig. 10 (A,B) Neuron density versus distance from electrode track for the non-stimulated and stimulated cats. (C,D) Glial cell density versus distance from electrode track for the non-stimulated and stimulated cats. Includes mean across all animals (4 non-stimulated, 4 stimulated), SD bars, and asterisks above the implanted/stimulated mean values that were significantly different from the control values ($p=<\alpha/2$, $\alpha=0.5$, Bonferroni multiplicity adjustment). Taken from Lenarz et al.[20] and reprinted with permission from Lippincott Williams & Wilkins.

track. Furthermore, it appears that chronic stimulation improved the tissue reaction (i.e. less glial cells relative to control) and led to better survival of the neurons around the electrode array. Further studies need to be performed to confirm this finding since it is based on only a few animals.

Overall, these histomorphological findings demonstrated that minimal neuronal damage occurs around the electrode array due to chronic implantation and stimulation of the implant. These results are similar to what has been observed with other neural implants currently used in human patients[21,22] and are encouraging as to the potential safety of our array for clinical use.

SURGICAL APPROACH

Considering that NF2 patients are the largest initial group of candidates for an AMI, the next step was to develop a combined surgical approach that enables removal of acoustic neuromas and AMI implantation at the same surgical setting. The typical midline and paramedian approaches both provide good exposure of the IC but do not provide an appropriate lateral exposure to the CPA and internal auditory canal, which is necessary for tumour removal. However, the lateral suboccipital craniotomy provides access to the internal auditory canal and CPA as well as the IC via a lateral supracerebellar–infratentorial approach (Fig. 11A,B). With regard to vestibular schwannoma surgery, this approach enables removal of even large tumours with the possibility of hearing preservation in patients who undergo surgery in the last hearing ear. In these cases, the function of the auditory nerve must

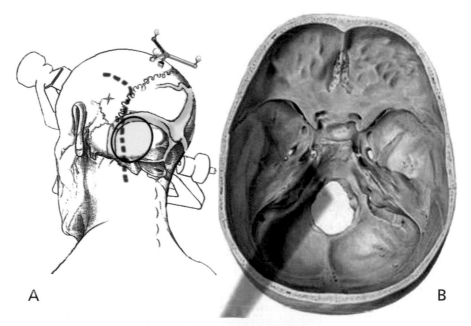

A

B

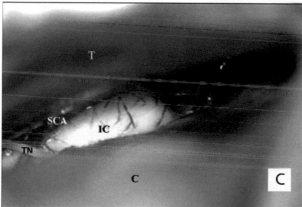

C

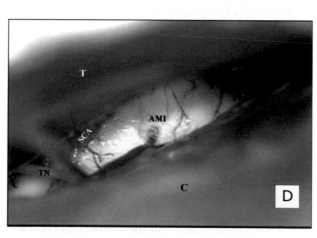

D

Fig. 11 (A) Schematic drawing showing the skin incision (red dotted line), appropriate location for the receiver-stimulator of the AMI in the tempo-parietal area (red star) and the location of the lateral suboccipital crani-otomy (yellow circle) exposing the inferior margin of the transverse sinus and the medial margin of the sigmoid sinus. (B) A schematic drawing showing the area of exposure provided by the lateral suboccipital craniotomy including the ipsilateral cerebello-pontine angle and the dorsolateral aspect of the mesencephalon. (C) Expo-sure of the left IC, troch-lear nerve (TN), and the caudal branch of the superior cerebellar artery (SCA) through the lateral supracerebellar–infratento rial approach. (D) A view of the AMI electrode array implanted into the IC in a fresh cadaver specimen. C, cerebellum; T, tentorium. Taken from Samii et al.[6] and reprinted with per-mission from Lippincott Williams & Wilkins.

43

be monitored during and after tumour removal, in which implantation would only be performed in the case of complete hearing loss.

We performed a series of anatomical dissections on fresh human cadavers in the semi-sitting position[6] and observed that approaching the tentorial hiatus and dorsolateral aspect of the mesencephalon through the lateral supracerebellar–infratentorial route does not endanger the major midline venous structures in the quadrigeminal cistern. It also provides direct access to the IC with an appropriate angle for AMI insertion along the hypothesised tonotopic gradient of the ICC (Fig. 11C,D). Potential risks of this combined approach are partly related to tumour removal through the typical lateral suboccipital approach in the semi-sitting position and partly due to the supracerebellar–infratentorial approach to the IC.[23–26] In experienced hands, tumour removal through this approach is associated with no mortality and a low rate of minor complications.[27] Using intra-operative Doppler sonography allows early detection, and thereby exclusion, of additional morbidity due to air embolism. Risks regarding exposure of the IC and AMI implantation include cerebellar bleeding or infarction, which may result from either extensive retraction of the cerebellum or from interruption or coagulation of the cerebellar bridging veins. In performing the operation in the semi-sitting position, there is no need for cerebellar retraction, and approaching the tentorial notch laterally helps in preserving the cerebellar bridging veins, which are mostly located medial to the trajectory of our approach. The major midline venous structures are not exposed and are, therefore, not in danger. The only cranial nerve surrounding the IC is the trochlear nerve, which emerges at the side of the frenulum veli below the IC and encircles the cerebral peduncle. Exposing this nerve immediately after opening the arachnoid adhesions reduces the risk for accidental damage to the nerve (Fig. 11C). Also, swelling of the superior colliculus either because of manipulation in the quadrigeminal cistern or inevitable coagulation of the quadrigeminal veins may lead to a transient Parinaud syndrome, consisting of a combination of impaired extra-ocular movements (impaired up-gaze or convergence), nystagmus, and impaired papillary reactions. These deficits are almost always transient and rarely cause permanent neurological sequelae.[28]

CLINICAL FINDINGS IN THE FIRST THREE PATIENTS

SURGICAL RESULTS

The AMI clinical study was conducted in accordance with ISO 14155 (International Standard for Clinical Investigation of Medical Devices) and follows the Good Clinical Practice guidelines. Medical Ethics Committee and Competent Authority written approvals according to national laws were obtained and patients signed informed consent forms prior to AMI implantation and testing.

Currently, three NF2 patients have been implanted with the AMI array. All three patients required acoustic neuroma removal on one side where they were already deaf. Extensive pre-operative audiological testing was performed to confirm neural deafness on the selected side. The 3-D navigation CT and MRI images based on the fixed bone anchored registration method were used for intra-operative navigation and identification of the right angle for electrode insertion. In all three patients, removal of the acoustic neuroma and AMI implantation were performed at the same surgical setting through the lateral suboccipital–supracerebellar–infratentorial approach as explained above. The goal was to perform a surgical approach that enabled tumour removal and then AMI implantation with minimal added complications. The implantation was performed by a multidisciplinary team composed of neurosurgeons, otolaryngologists, and electrophysiologists. Intra-operative monitoring of the facial nerve was performed during tumour removal and of the trochlear nerve during AMI implantation. Electrically evoked middle latency responses to AMI stimulation were also assessed to confirm proper placement in the auditory midbrain. Due to the semi-sitting approach, precordial Doppler monitoring was performed throughout the operation. The amount of time required for exposure of the IC and AMI implantation for our experienced neurosurgeons was comparable to the time required for exposure of the lateral recess of the 4th ventricle and ABI implantation.

None of the patients developed any complications either due to tumour removal or AMI implantation. There were no transient or permanent sensory or motor deficits due to the implantation trauma in the midbrain. Also, none of the patients experienced transient or permanent pain sensations postoperatively due to potential lesions in the midbrain. Using 3-D CT images fused with the pre-operative 3 D MRI images (for details, see Lim et al.[29]), we were able to identify the location of the array within the midbrain immediately after the operation as well as 4 weeks later after brain alterations due to surgery (e.g. associated with swelling and excess air) subsided. Our experience

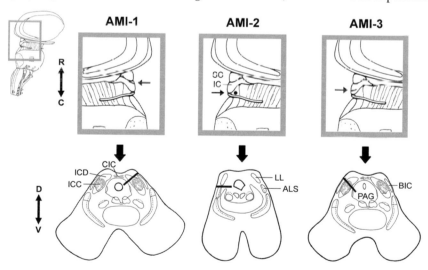

Fig. 12 Parasagittal (top) and axial (bottom) sections showing the location and orientation of the array within the midbrain of each patient. Arrow in parasagittal section points to the caudorostral location of the array and the corresponding axial section below. The black line (or dot for AMI-2) representing the array in each section corresponds to the trajectory of the array across several superimposed CT-MRI slices. ALS, anterolateral system; BIC, brachium of IC; CIC, commissure of IC; IC, inferior colliculus; ICC, inferior colliculus central nucleus; ICD, inferior colliculus dorsal cortex; LL, lateral lemniscus; PAG, periaqueductal grey; SC, superior colliculus. Taken from Lim et al.[29] and reprinted with permission from the Society for Neuroscience.

with ABI patients showed that the most probable time period for electrode migration is the first 4 weeks after implantation. None of our patients showed evidence of electrode dislocation.

Figure 12 provides the location of the implanted AMI array in each patient based on the CT–MRI reconstructions. Due to our learning experience with the surgical approach, the array was not implanted into the intended target of the ICC in the first two patients. AMI-1 was implanted into the dorsal region of the IC, while AMI-2 was implanted on the surface of the lateral lemniscus. With improvements in our surgical techniques, we were able to position the array into the ICC in AMI-3. The fortuitous outcome of these different placements is that we were able to assess the effects of stimulation within various midbrain regions on auditory activation and perception.

The first fitting was performed 4 weeks after implantation in each patient. Stimulation of the AMI sites produced both auditory and non-auditory effects. The non-auditory sensations consisted mostly of sensory effects associated with paresthesia in different parts of the body. None of the stimulated sites elicited any pain sensations or blood pressure and heart rate changes as might be expected from stimulation of deeper midbrain regions. All non-auditory sites were turned off for daily use. Details of these side-effects and their corresponding stimulated regions will be presented in a separate publication.

PSYCHOPHYSICAL RESULTS

All three patients obtained various loudness, temporal, pitch, and directional percepts with stimulation of their AMI sites. A detailed description of these effects are presented elsewhere[29] and only a brief overview is presented here. As mentioned above, some sites elicited non-auditory percepts and were turned off for psychophysical testing and daily use. However, for the active sites, the patients described the percepts as tonal in nature but that some sites elicited a broad spectral percept with multiple pitches, which occurred most frequently in AMI-2 whose sites appear to be located outside the IC acting as surface electrodes. The patients also described the sounds as having an electronic quality mixed in with the tonal percept. What was interesting is that each patient perceived the sounds as originating from a different location. Stimulation of all sites in AMI-1 elicited binaural percepts in which the loudness varied between sides. For AMI-2, all sounds originated from the ipsilateral side, while for AMI-3 all sounds originated from the contralateral side. The binaural effects observed in AMI-1 could be caused by activation of binaural pathways within the dorsal cortex of the IC.[30] The monaural effects observed in AMI-2 and AMI-3 support the existence of segregated sound localisation pathways projecting through the ventral portion of the lateral lemniscus and the dorsomedial region of the ICC, respectively.[31–33]

Figure 13 summarises the T- and C-levels measured for different sites in each patient over time as the patients continued to use their implant on a daily basis. The T- and C-levels for AMI-1 continued to rise reaching the compliance voltage of our stimulator (at +125 days). Due to this rise in levels, we turned off the processor for 48 days to assess if values would return to usable levels. The activation levels decreased dramatically, but not completely to the initial values. It is not clear as to what may be causing these adaptive effects. One

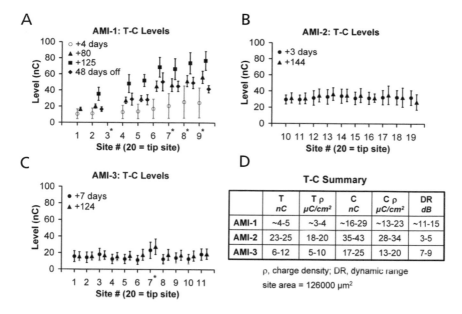

Fig. 13 Threshold (T) and comfortable (C) levels measured in each patient using 500 ms on-off pulse trains with 250 pps, 100 μs/phase monopolar pulses. (A) T- and C-levels (end-points of bar) for AMI-1 measured for four different time points (symbols) from when the implant was initially turned on. Due to rising levels over time, the implant was turned off for 48 days (after the +125-day measurement) and then T- and C-levels were measured again. At +4 days, only the modified T- and C-levels used for the daily processor rather than the actual measured values were available. Thus they are labelled with an open symbol and lighter shaded bars. (B,C) T- and C-levels for AMI-2 and AMI-3 measured at two different time points and demonstrating stability over time. (D) Summary of values for each patient only for the values from the first testing session shown in (A–C). Asterisks correspond to sites shorted to other inactive sites, except for site 3 (shorted to active site 9) for AMI-1, that were turned off. Taken from Lim et al.[29] and reprinted with permission from the Society for Neuroscience.

hypothesis is that the stimulation rates and patterns are overdriving the neurons located within the dorsal IC region, which receives a large number of projections from auditory and non-auditory centres[34] and may be designed for adapting to different stimuli.[35] We are currently investigating various stimulation strategies for effective and stable activation. The other two patients exhibited stable activation levels over time (Fig. 13B,C) suggesting that location of stimulation, thus the type of neurons activated, is important for AMI implementation. The auditory sensations and/or side-effects associated with each site have generally remained stable indicating minimal movement of the implant over time.

Particularly for AMI-3 who is implanted within the ICC, it is interesting that the thresholds were not lower (6–12 nC; Fig. 13D) than those observed for cochlear implant patients (5–20 nC)[36,37] as was predicted from our animal results. However, this may be explained by recent findings by Lim and Anderson[19] showing that stimulation of more caudal and dorsal regions along the isofrequency laminae of the ICC, where AMI-3 is implanted, can require current levels more than 17 dB compared to more rostral and ventral regions

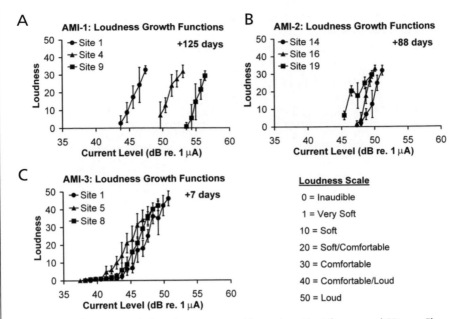

Fig. 14 Loudness growth functions measured in each patient (mean and SD; *n* = 5) using 500 ms bursts with 250 pps, 100 µs/phase monopolar pulses. Taken from Lim *et al.*[29] and reprinted with permission from the Society for Neuroscience.

for cortical activation. AMI-2 was implanted on the surface of the lateral lemniscus, which would explain the higher current levels to activate more distant auditory neurons.

Several psychophysical features have been shown to be important for speech perception performance, including loudness coding, spectral discrimination, and temporal acuity.[11,38,39,46,47] Figure 14 demonstrates that all three patients obtain loudness growth functions that monotonically increased with current level. It is interesting that we observed a shallow loudness growth tail for lower current levels in AMI-3, which may be related to the location of stimulation within the midbrain. It is also possible that the other two patients were less able to detect soft sounds at lower current levels, especially for AMI-2 who had stronger tinnitus effects.

In terms of spectral coding, we tested the patients' ability to pitch order their sites using several different methods (*i.e.* pitch ranking use a 2-AFC paradigm, pitch scaling, and absolute pitch assessment). If the ICC consists of a well-defined tonotopic structure[7,9,12] and frequency-specific stimulation is achievable based on our animal results presented above, then it is expected that stimulation within an isofrequency lamina should elicit a specific pitch percept that changes systematically (*i.e.* low to high) with location (*i.e.* towards deeper ICC regions) as occurs with cochlear stimulation. However, we did not observe any systematic shift in pitch, particularly in AMI-3 whose array is supposedly aligned along the tonotopic gradient of the ICC. Different pitches were perceived and a few sites consistently elicited higher or lower pitches. However, there were fluctuations in pitch percepts across most of the sites over time and even within the same day. Furthermore, stimulation of all the active sites in each patient elicited predominantly low-pitch percepts with none eliciting a high-pitch percept (*i.e.* lower than a woman's voice). It is possible that location of midbrain stimulation, especially along the isofrequency dimension of the ICC, can affect the extent of frequency-specific activation and the elicited pitch percept. It is also possible that long-term deafness effects (AMI–3 was deaf for 6 years) may have compromised coding properties within the central auditory system. Recent and dramatic improvements in various coding properties, including pitch and speech perception in AMI-3 (results will be presented in a future publication) suggest plasticity plays an important role in AMI implementation.

We have also performed several temporal tests, such as gap detection, modulation detection, and pulse rate tests to determine how well our patients can detect fine changes in the temporal structure of the stimuli. These results will be presented in future publications. The main findings are that each patient can detect changes in temporal patterns of stimulation and the extent of this temporal acuity appears to depend on location of stimulation within the midbrain.

SPEECH RESULTS

Each patient received several days of speech and environmental sound training during the first week the implant was turned on. The patients returned for several days every month so we could adjust their processors, perform various psychophysical tests and training sessions, and assess their speech perception performance. We used traditional cochlear implant stimulation strategies (AMI-1, ACE; AMI-2, SPEAK; AMI-3, SPEAK; Cochlear Ltd), which are the only ones currently approved for our AMI patients. Basic parameters that need to be set for these algorithms include the T- and C-levels, pulse rate, pulse width, electrode configuration, and site ordering. We decided to use a pulse rate of 250 pps, pulse width of 100 μs/phase, and monopolar (MP1+2) configuration. These parameters were selected based on various psychophysical tests and will be presented in a future publication. Briefly, 250 pps was high enough to avoid noticeable rate pitch effects (*i.e.* increasing rates up to 2900 pps did not noticably increase the pith from that at 250 pps) and the lowest rate available for daily stimulation to minimise adaptive effects. These parameters also achieved the largest drop in thresholds in which using longer pulse widths and higher pulse rates (thus greater total charge) did not decease thresholds by much more, whereas using shorter pulse widths and slower pulse rates substantially increased threshold levels. This was important for ensuring effective activation within the compliance voltage limits of the stimulator. The T- and C-levels as well as the site (*i.e.* pitch) order was adjusted as needed during each testing session.

All methods for the speech tests are presented elsewhere[29,40] and were performed in live voice under lip-reading alone (V), lip reading plus the AMI (VA), and AMI alone (A). The difference between lip-reading plus AMI and lip-reading alone is known as lip-reading enhancement. Figure 15 summarises the results for all three patients for the vowel, consonant, number, and speech tracking tests at 6 months of use. For the vowel test, all three patients achieved high scores for lip-reading alone making it difficult to detect significant lip-reading enhancement with the AMI. However, AMI-2 and AMI-3 obtained 23%

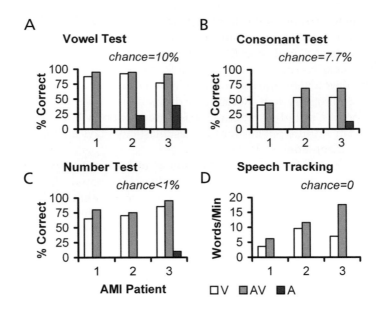

Fig. 15 Speech test scores at 6 months. Vowel test (chance level of 10%) consisted of 5 long (*e.g.* BAAT, GAAT) and 5 short (*e.g.* BAT, GAT) words randomly read to the patient (4 times) and the patient had to repeat the word. Consonant test (chance level of 7.7%) consisted of 13 meaningless consonant words (*e.g.* ABA, AGA) repeated 4 times. Freiburger number test (open set, chance level < 1%) consisted of 20 German numbers between 13 and 99 (2–5 syllables). Speech tracking (modified open set, chance level of 0%) involved reading a story to the patient who was asked to repeat the words of the cited sentences. The number of correct words in 5 min was obtained and divided by 5 to obtain the correct number of words per minute. V, lip-reading (visual) alone; AV, lip-reading and AMI (audiovisual); A, AMI (audio) alone. Lip-reading enhancement is the difference between AV and V. A value of 0 means we could not test. Taken from Lim et al.[29] and reprinted with permission from the Society for Neuroscience.

and 40% correct (10% chance level), respectively, with the AMI alone indicating that they are obtaining some speech information with their implants. For the consonant and number tests, only AMI-3 performed above chance with the AMI alone (12.5% and 10%, respectively). Chance level is 7.7% for the consonant test and less than 1% for the number test. AMI-3 also partially identified the different numbers 55% of the time under AMI alone (*e.g.* stated twenty-two for twenty-three). Furthermore, all three patients exhibited some lip-reading enhancement with the AMI. Figure 8D presents speech tracking results. Under lip-reading alone, the patients achieved about 4–10 words per minute. For both AMI and lip-reading, they obtained a lip-reading enhancement of about 2–11 words per minute (chance level of 0). These speech results in the AMI patients, particularly for AMI-3 who is implanted in the intended target (ICC), are comparable to those observed in ABI NF2 patients that were tested at 6 months in the same clinic using the same protocol.[40]

Overall, the patients are benefiting from their implants on a daily basis. They have all experienced improvements in their awareness of environmental sounds, such as cars driving by, birds chirping, doors shutting, and the telephone ringing. We have observed the most rapid improvements in AMI-3, who is implanted in the intended target of the ICC. The other two patients are improving more slowly due to their dependence on residual hearing and the location of their implants. Prior to implantation, AMI-3 was completely dependent on written conversation and had difficulties in controlling the volume of her voice. She is now able to speak at a consistent loudness level, has improved the articulation of words, and no longer depends on written conversations.

SUMMARY

The AMI has potential as an alternative hearing solution for patients who cannot benefit from cochlear implants. Our electrophysiological and histomorphological findings in animals demonstrated that ICC stimulation can achieve effective activation of the auditory pathways and with minimal damage to neurons surrounding the implanted AMI array. These findings, along with the development of a safe surgical approach, enabled us to pursue clinical trials. In the first three implanted patients, we demonstrated that the AMI is safe for human use and provides different loudness, pitch, temporal, and directional percepts, features that have shown to be important for speech perception[11,38,39,46,47] and more complex sound processing.[41-43] Furthermore, the AMI thus far provides performance levels comparable to the ABI in NF2 patients, particularly for patient AMI-3 who is the only patient implanted in the intended region, the ICC. Considering that the IC is more surgically exposable than the cochlear nucleus, this argues for the use of the AMI as a potential alternative to the ABI. However, it is important that we properly place the array into the ICC. Due to our learning experience with the surgical approach, the array was not implanted into the intended target in the first two patients, which limited their overall performance. With recent improvements in our surgical techniques, we should be able to implant the array within appropriate regions within the ICC and enable better performance levels as was observed for AMI-3.

The question remains as to how we can improve performance in our current and future patients. Currently, we are using simple stimulation strategies originally designed for cochlear implant patients. This, along with the short period of training, is partly why our patients have only achieved moderate improvements in hearing. It is expected that with greater training and with more appropriate stimuli, speech perception performance should improve. Furthermore, based on our recent human findings (unpublished observation) and animal results,[19] stimulation of different regions within the ICC affect various sound coding properties. For example, stimulation of more rostral and ventral regions along the isofrequency dimension of the ICC elicit enhanced temporal precision, greater spatial synchronisation, greater neural activation, and better level coding. Thus, implanting an array within these regions may improve overall hearing performance compared to that of AMI-3, who is implanted into a more caudal and dorsal region. On the other hand, it may be that an optimal region for our single shank array does not exist and we will need to activate multiple regions simultaneously across the frequency and isofrequency dimensions of the ICC to elicit the desired percept. These are all issues that we are currently investigating in our human patients and animal models. The hope is that we are able to first identify appropriate ICC regions for implantation and develop basic stimulation paradigms that can enable speech perception performance above what is observed in conventional ABI patients. The next step will be to develop more complex electrode technologies and stimuli to achieve higher levels of hearing, especially in noisy environments.

Key points for clinical practice

- Tumour-induced damage in the cochlear nucleus may be responsible for the limited success of the auditory brainstem implant (ABI) in neurofibromatosis type 2 (NF2) patients. Therefore, an alternative implantation site that bypasses the damaged pathways in the brainstem may provide better hearing performance in NF2 patients.

- The central nucleus of the inferior colliculus provides access to almost all ascending auditory information and has a well-defined tonotopic organisation which is important for an auditory prosthesis.

- The auditory midbrain implant is a single-shank multi-electrode array designed according to the dimensions of the human inferior colliculus with the goal of stimulating the different frequency layers of its central nucleus.

- Animal experiments show that the auditory midbrain implant (AMI) is able to achieve frequency specific activation of the inferior colliculus within safe limits for electrical stimulation of the central nervous system.

- Histomorphological evaluation of chronically implanted cats revealed intact and healthy neurons around the AMI array tracks in both stimulated and non-stimulated animals.

- A modified lateral suboccipital craniotomy provides access to the internal auditory canal and cerebellopontine angle as well as the inferior colliculus via a lateral supracerebellar–infratentorial approach, thus enables the removal of acoustic neuromas and AMI implantation in one surgical setting.

- AMI implantation can be safely performed at the same surgical setting after tumour removal. None of the three implanted NF2 patients developed any complications due to AMI implantation and stimulation.

- AMI provides different loudness, pitch, temporal, and directional percepts. However, the results strongly depend on the location of the electrode array in the midbrain.

- All three patients experienced improvements in their awareness of environmental sounds and their lip-reading abilities. The greatest improvement was observed in the third patient in whom the array is located in the intended target of the inferior colliculus central nucleus.

- With correct placement of the electrode array within the central nucleus of the inferior colliculus and appropriate stimulation strategies, the AMI may provide a better alternative for hearing restoration in NF2 patients than the conventional ABI.

References

1. Hitselberger WE, House WF, Edgerton BJ *et al*. Cochlear nucleus implants. *Otolaryngol Head Neck Surg* 1984; **92**: 52–54.
2. Lenarz T. Cochlear implants: what can be achieved? *Am J Otol* 1997; **18**: S2–S3.
3. Lenarz T. Cochlear implants: selection criteria and shifting borders. *Acta Otorhinolaryngol Belg* 1998; **52**: 183–199.
4. Adams JS, Hasenstab MS, Pippin GW *et al*. Telephone use and understanding in patients with cochlear implants. *Ear Nose Throat J* 2004; **83**: 96, 9–100, 2–3.
5. Colletti V, Shannon RV. Open set speech perception with auditory brainstem implant? *Laryngoscope* 2005; **115**: 1974–1978.
6. Samii A, Lenarz M, Majdani O *et al*. Auditory midbrain implant: a combined approach for vestibular schwannoma surgery and device implantation. *Otol Neurotol* 2007; **28**: 31–38.
7. Geniec P, Morest DK. The neuronal architecture of the human posterior colliculus. A study with the Golgi method. *Acta Otolaryngol Suppl* 1971; **295**: 1–33.
8. Moore JK. The human auditory brain stem: a comparative view. *Hear Res* 1987; **29**: 1–32.
9. Oliver DL. Neuronal organization in the inferior colliculus. In: Winer JA, Schreiner CE. (eds) *The Inferior Colliculus*. New York: Springer Science+Business Media, 2005; 69–114.
10. Casseday JH, Fremouw T, Covey E. The inferior colliculus: a hub for the central auditory system. In: Oertel D, Fay RR, Popper AN. (eds) *Springer Handbook of Auditory Research: Integrative Functions in the Mammalian Auditory Pathway*, vol. 15). New York: Springer, 2002; 238–318.
11. Friesen LM, Shannon RV, Baskent D *et al*. Speech recognition in noise as a function of the number of spectral channels: comparison of acoustic hearing and cochlear implants. *J Acoust Soc Am* 2001; **110**: 1150–1163.
12. Schreiner CE, Langner G. Laminar fine structure of frequency organization in auditory midbrain. *Nature* 1997; **388**: 383–386.
13. Lenarz T, Lim HH, Reuter G *et al*. The auditory midbrain implant: a new auditory prosthesis for neural deafness-concept and device description. *Otol Neurotol* 2006; **27**: 838–843.
14. Lenarz M, Lim HH, Patrick JF *et al*. Electrophysiological validation of a human prototype auditory midbrain implant in a guinea pig model. *JARO* 2006; **7**: 383–398.
15. Bierer JA, Middlebrooks JC. Auditory cortical images of cochlear-implant stimuli: dependence on electrode configuration. *J Neurophysiol* 2002; **87**: 478–492.
16. McCreery DB, Agnew WF, Yuen TG *et al*. Charge density and charge per phase as cofactors in neural injury induced by electrical stimulation. *IEEE Trans Biomed Eng* 1990; **37**: 996–1001.
17. Shannon RV. A model of safe levels for electrical stimulation. *IEEE Trans Biomed Eng* 1992; **39**: 424–426.
18. Lim HH, Anderson DJ. Auditory cortical responses to electrical stimulation of the inferior colliculus: implications for an auditory midbrain implant. *J Neurophysiol* 2006; **96**: 975–988.
19. Lim HH, Anderson DJ. Spatially distinct functional output regions within the central nucleus of the inferior colliculus: implications for an auditory midbrain implant. *J Neurosci* 2007; **27**: 8733–8743.
20. Lenarz M, Lim HH, Lenarz T *et al*. Auditory midbrain implant: histomorphological effects of long-term implantation and electrical stimulation of a new DBS array. *Otol Neurotol* 2007; **28**: 1045–1052.
21. Haberler C, Alesch F, Mazal PR *et al*. No tissue damage by chronic deep brain stimulation in Parkinson's disease. *Ann Neurol* 2000; **48**: 372–376.
22. McCreery DB, Shannon RV, Otto S *et al*. A cochlear nucleus auditory prosthesis based on microstimulation, Quarterly Report #3, Contract NO1-DC-4-0005, National Institute on Deafness and Other Communication Disorders: Neural Prosthesis Development Program, 2005.
23. Vougioukas VI, Omran H, Glasker S *et al*. Far lateral supracerebellar infratentorial approach for the treatment of upper brainstem gliomas: clinical experience with pediatric patients. *Childs Nerv Syst* 2005; **21**: 1037–1041.
24. Ulm AJ, Tanriover N, Kawashima M *et al*. Microsurgical approaches to the perimesencephalic cisterns and related segments of the posterior cerebral artery: comparison using a novel application of image guidance. *Neurosurgery* 2004; **54**: 1313–1327, discussion 27–28.
25. Hitotsumatsu T, Matsushima T, Inoue T. Microvascular decompression for treatment of trigeminal neuralgia, hemifacial spasm, and glossopharyngeal neuralgia: three surgical approach variations. *Neurosurgery* 2003; **53**: 1436–1441, discussion 42–43.

26. Ammirati M, Bernardo A, Musumeci A *et al*. Comparison of different infratentorial-supracerebellar approaches to the posterior and middle incisural space: a cadaveric study. *J Neurosurg* 2002; **97**: 922–928.

27. Samii M, Gerganov V, Samii A. Improved preservation of hearing and facial nerve function in vestibular schwannoma surgery via the retrosigmoid approach in a series of 200 patients. *J Neurosurg* 2006; **105**: 527–535.

28. Stein BM. Supracerebellar-infratentorial approach to pineal tumors. *Surg Neurol* 1979; **11**: 331–337.

29. Lim HH, Lenarz T, Joseph G *et al*. Electrical stimulation of the midbrain for hearing restoration: insight into the functional organization of the human central auditory system. *J Neurosci* 2007; 27: 13541–13551.

30. Saldana E, Merchan MA. Intrinsic and commissural connections of the inferior colliculus. In: Winer JA, Schreiner CE. (eds) *The Inferior Colliculus*. New York: Springer Science+Business Media, 2005; 155–181.

31. Oliver DL. Projections to the inferior colliculus from the anteroventral cochlear nucleus in the cat: possible substrates for binaural interaction. *J Comp Neurol* 1987; **264**: 24–46.

32. Schofield BR. Superior olivary complex and lateral lemniscal connections of the auditory midbrain. In: Winer JA, Schreiner CE. (eds) *The Inferior Colliculus*. New York: Springer Science+Business Media, 2005; 132–154.

33. Loftus WC, Bishop DC, Saint Marie RL *et al*. Organization of binaural excitatory and inhibitory inputs to the inferior colliculus from the superior olive. *J Comp Neurol* 2004; **472**: 330–344.

34. Winer JA. Three systems of descending projections to the inferior colliculus. In: Winer JA, Schreiner CE. (eds) *The Inferior Colliculus*. New York: Springer Science+Business Media, 2005; 231–247.

35. Perez-Gonzalez D, Malmierca MS, Covey E. Novelty detector neurons in the mammalian auditory midbrain. *Eur J Neurosci* 2005; **22**: 2879–2885.

36. Pfingst BE, Zwolan TA, Holloway LA. Effects of stimulus configuration on psychophysical operating levels and on speech recognition with cochlear implants. *Hear Res* 1997; **112**: 247–260.

37. Shannon RV. Threshold and loudness functions for pulsatile stimulation of cochlear implants. *Hear Res* 1985; **18**: 135–143.

38. Shannon RV, Zeng FG, Kamath V *et al*. Speech recognition with primarily temporal cues. *Science* 1995; **270**: 303–304.

39. Nelson DA, Schmitz JL, Donaldson GS *et al*. Intensity discrimination as a function of stimulus level with electric stimulation. *J Acoust Soc Am* 1996; **100**: 2393–2414.

40. Lenarz T, Moshrefi M, Matthies C *et al*. Auditory brainstem implant: part I. Auditory performance and its evolution over time. *Otol Neurotol* 2001; **22**: 823–833.

41. Smith ZM, Delgutte B, Oxenham AJ. Chimaeric sounds reveal dichotomies in auditory perception. *Nature* 2002; **416**: 87–90.

42. Shannon RV, Fu QJ, Galvin 3rd J. The number of spectral channels required for speech recognition depends on the difficulty of the listening situation. *Acta Otolaryngol Suppl* 2004: 50–54.

43. Kidd Jr G, Arbogast TL, Mason CR *et al*. The advantage of knowing where to listen. *J Acoust Soc Am* 2005; **118**: 3804–3815.

44. Malmierca MS, Rees A, Le Beau FE *et al*. Laminar organization of frequency-defined local axons within and between the inferior colliculi of the guinea pig. *J Comp Neurol* 1995; **357**: 124–144.

45. Wallace MN, Rutkowski RG, Palmer AR. Identification and localisation of auditory areas in guinea pig cortex. *Exp Brain Res* 2000; **132**: 445–456.

46. Loizou PC, Dorman M, Fitzke J. The effect of reduced dynamic range on speech understanding: implications for patients with cochlear implants. *Ear Hear* 2000; **21**: 25–31.

47. Zeng FG, Galvin 3rd JJ. Amplitude mapping and phoneme recognition in cochlear listeners. *Ear Hear* 1999; **20**: 60–74.

Joachim Müller

4

Bilateral cochlear implantation

Binaural hearing, our ability to hear with two ears, is essential to cope with a variety of every-day listening situations.[1] Satisfactory auditory quality, improved speech understanding in noise, directional hearing, source separation and spatial hearing require two ears. Some hearing tasks can, indeed, only be mastered with two ears. The best-known example is localisation of a sound source. However, binaural hearing is not only important for localisation but fulfils various other hearing tasks, such as separation of sound sources, suppression of sound coloration and improved speech understanding in noise.[1]

BINAURAL HEARING

SPATIAL HEARING

As mentioned above, binaural hearing is essential for spatial hearing. As natural as it may seem to us today that two ears are necessary for sound localisation, this aspect has been considered an important fact only since the experiments done by the physiologist Ernst Heinrich Weber (1795–1858).[2]

INTERAURAL LEVEL AND TIME DIFFERENCES, HEAD SHADOW EFFECT

The ability to localise a sound source depends mainly on three effects:

1. Linear distortion caused by deflection and reflection at body, head and, most of all, the auricular recesses. They enable differentiation between up/down and front/back.

Joachim Müller MD PhD
Assistant Professor at Department of Otolaryngology, Head and Neck Surgery at the University of Würzburg, Klinik und Poliklinik für Hals-, Nasen- und Ohrenkranke der Universität, Josef-Schneider-Strasse 11, 97080 Würzburg, Germany
E-mail: joachim.m@mail.uni-wuerzburg.de

2. Analysis of time differences in the horizontal plane.

3. Analysis of level differences. Sound approaching from the right reaches the right ear a little sooner than the left ear. In addition, sound intensity is slightly higher in the right ear than the left ear because the head forms an obstacle for the sound wave, leaving the farther side of the head in a sound shadow.

LOCATION OF SOUND SOURCES, PRECEDENCE EFFECT

Beside localisation, binaural hearing allows estimation of the distance to a sound source. Localising sound sources in closed rooms requires special abilities because the sound emitted by a source reaches the ear differently – directly and after several reflections from walls and other reverberant objects.

Although sound reaching the ears takes various pathways, no echo is heard in small rooms. All reflections merge into one auditory perception. The auditory system can even localise the source of complex sounds such as speech or music. It is mainly determined by the first sound wave front reaching the ear. This phenomenon is known as the 'precedence effect'.

IMPROVED HEARING IN NOISE: BMLD, BILD

Another phenomenon is closely connected with binaural hearing: differences in the signals in both ears reduce the masking effect of noise. In contrast to hearing with only one ear, or when presenting diotic signals, dichotic test signals are heard at softer volumes although the noise level remains the same. This effect is known as 'binaural masking level difference' (BMLD) and is observed when signal and noise source are differently localised in space. When using speech signals, we talk about 'binaural intelligibility level difference' (BILD).

COCKTAIL PARTY PHENOMENON

Hellbrück[2] considers BMLD and BILD effects as closely related to the cocktail party phenomenon. The cocktail party effect describes the interesting observation that it is possible to select an individual speaker from a babble of voices. Monaural hearing reduces this ability significantly so that a functional binaural system seems to be necessary to suppress noise.

AUDITORY PATTERN RECOGNITION, RECOGNISING THE ENVIRONMENT

Beside the ability to localise acoustic events in 3-dimensional space, it is also possible to identify such events, *e.g.* to differentiate and recognise musical instruments. We recognise people by their voices in various listening situations. We are even able to distinguish individual voices in a babble of voices.[2] In addition, binaural hearing is important for acoustically recognising the environment and, in conjunction with the visual and haptic sense, for the mental representation of the environment (Merzenich, Jenkins and Middlebrooks, cited after Hellbrück[2]).

BILATERAL COCHLEAR IMPLANTATION

A BRIEF HISTORY

First results with a bilaterally implanted patient in Australia in the early 1990s were not very encouraging.[3,4] Although fusion of the auditory perception of both implants was obtained, speech understanding was not significantly improved.[3] After these discouraging results, the Australian group did not continue with binaural cochlear implantation to improve hearing for years.

In 1996, the group in Würzburg were the first world-wide to succeed in significantly improving a patient's speech understanding in quiet and in noise and to restore directional hearing only 4 weeks after first fitting.[5]

Following the first positive results in adults, children have been binaurally implanted since 1998. In 1999, these early and convincing results were presented to a large scientific community as an announced discussion, hoping for a lasting improvement for many more children.[6]

Animal experiments have proven the neuroprotective effect of electrical stimulation on the auditory nerve[7] and the development of the auditory pathway. When implanting the first children, it was not clear if and how these children might benefit from the second implant; however, considering the encouraging results in adults and by analogy to normal hearing and hearing aid use, it was quite sensible to assume that children would benefit from binaural hearing.

IMPROVED SPEECH UNDERSTANDING IN QUIET AND IN NOISE

Bilateral implant users benefit from lasting improvement of speech understanding in quiet and in noise (~20% better speech understanding in quiet in the Freiburg monosyllables; ~30% better speech understanding in the HSM sentences in noise).[8–11] The effects and improved speech understanding in quiet and in noise observed in adults were also proven for children.[9] Meanwhile, the Würzburg results have been confirmed in other studies. When assessing binaural improvement, we must bear in mind that the binaural hearing condition is compared with the better ear, not with the worse ear. Bilateral implantation undeniably supplies the better ear which is not necessarily the case in unilateral implantations. Diagnosing the ear with the better postoperative results before implantation remains difficult and for many individuals nearly impossible.

(RE-)ESTABLISHING DIRECTIONAL AND SPATIAL HEARING

Binaural hearing enables spatial hearing, directional hearing and the separation of sound sources. To evaluate bilateral cochlear implant users' ability to localise, localisation experiments were conducted and the influence of interaural time and level differences analysed. Eight of nine subjects were able to localise and analyse interaural level and time differences. Bilateral users benefit from the known effects of binaural hearing just like individuals with normal hearing: head shadow effect, squelch effect and binaural summation effects.[10,11,20,23,24]

It was exciting to see if binaurally implanted children developed spatial and directional hearing. In her MD thesis, C. Edelmann observed the first 13 bilaterally implanted children over a period of 3 years. She found that directional hearing developed at different rates. It took an average time of 1.5 years before the children developed directional hearing. Over a period of 3 years, the children not only developed directional hearing but their misjudging directions decreased with increasing binaural hearing experience. Obviously, the children learn to localise a sound source in space and also learn to localise this sound source more accurately. Recent publications by Litowski and colleagues[18,19] confirm these results. Directional hearing in individuals with normal hearing depends on using interaural time and level differences and on deflection phenomena and reflection of sound at the auricle. Like individuals with normal hearing, bilateral cochlear implant users benefit from the same access to time and level differences.[10]

BILATERAL COCHLEAR IMPLANTATION AFTER MENINGITIS

In cases of meningitis, which may lead to partial or complete obliteration of both cochleae so that the electrode cannot be placed inside the cochlea at a later time, it is important to act quickly. Implanting both sides at the same surgical intervention is indicated unless severe medical reasons contra-indicate such an approach.

SIMULTANEOUS OR SEQUENTIAL IMPLANTATION

This question is still controversially discussed among experts and cannot yet be fully answered. The discussion deals with medical problems (anaesthesia in children, blood loss, surgical technique, *etc.*), aspects of development and maturation of hearing (sensitive periods for speech and language acquisition, development phases of binaural hearing), economical aspects (costs, personnel costs, *etc.*) and aspects of rehabilitation (training requirements for second side, *etc.*).

As our experience during the last decade has shown, children learn to hear with both implanted ears independently of whether they received their implants simultaneously or sequentially. General neurophysiological considerations lead to the assumption that binaural hearing develops faster and is more balanced in cases of simultaneous implantation. However, after 10 years of experience, we know that not only simultaneously implanted children but also sequentially implanted children benefit from binaural hearing. Sequential implantation with a longer interval in between the two surgeries (*i.e.* longer than 2 years) is not necessarily a disadvantage but requires special therapy considerations and training, particularly when the interval between the surgeries has been rather long. Children implanted sequentially with a short interval (*i.e.* shorter than 6–9 months) develop binaural hearing competence usually without additional special training. Considering the risks of a longer lasting simultaneous bilateral surgery (more than 4 h for both sides), sequential implantation with a short interval of 1 week between surgeries and with simultaneous first fitting may be a good compromise.

OPTIMAL TIME FOR BILATERAL IMPLANTATION

Based on experience and knowledge about the maturation of the auditory system (auditory nerve and auditory centres in the brain), it seems safe to assume that the sooner a child starts hearing with two ears, the better adapted the auditory pathways and the auditory centres will be and the less intensive bilateral hearing and speech/language therapy will have to be (see also Bauer et al.[14] and Shama et al.[15]).

Simultaneously implanted children need not train binaural hearing. The hearing sensations of both ears are integrated from the beginning. Training need increases the longer the interval between the surgeries. Implantation intervals of a few weeks up to several months seem desirable when it comes to training requirements. Longer intervals between implantations do not contra-indicate bilateral implantation. Children and teenagers benefit from binaural hearing despite longer intervals. In addition, a child's individual (learning) prerequisites (age, age at first implantation, possible residual hearing, [binaural] experience with hearing aids, general auditory and verbal development, etc.) play a role.

CONTRA-INDICATIONS FOR BILATERAL SUPPLY

The prerequisites for cochlear implantation must be assessed with examinations and medical diagnosis. Asymmetrical hearing, for instance, can be treated with a combination of a hearing aid on one side and a cochlear implant on the other. The benefit of bilateral cochlear implantation must be critically reviewed in such cases.

Unilateral malformation with an anatomically and morphologically normal cochlea on the contralateral side may indicate unilateral cochlear implantation. Older children and teenagers who are sufficiently mature and understanding should be included in the decision-making process to help them accept the second implant and any additionally necessary training. The child's lack of co-operation is a serious 'contra-indication'.

Unilateral loss of vestibular function bears a minimal risk of compromising residual vestibular function during surgery with possible consequences afterwards. Benefit of expected bilateral hearing must be weighed against this risk.

ETHICAL, ECONOMIC AND LEGAL CONSIDERATIONS

Denying children born deaf access to the hearing world for financial reasons claimed by social insurance is objectionable from a medical point of view. Considering the few cochlear implantations in our country, it is not ethically justifiable to withhold considerable improvement of their hearing situation from any patients. The total costs required for bilateral cochlear implantations are relatively small, particularly in relation to, for example, the general economic benefit. The obtained benefit exceeds by far the costs of implantation since children are given the opportunity to hear, thus improving their access to professional training and integration in the job market. An economically sound approach would be to keep working patients fit for work (keeping them also as tax payers and contributors to social security and insurance systems) by bilateral implantation, rather than retire them at the expense of social insurance.[12]

The lawyer B. Kochs has addressed legal aspects of bilateral cochlear implantation in several publications in the *Schnecke*.

The most difficult question of bilateral cochlear implantation is the one about elderly patients with higher risks of surgery and anaesthesia. If they desire bilateral implantation to improve their situation, they cannot possibly be denied as long as they are willing to bear the risks.

However, bilateral implantation does not lead to a 'post-implantation wave' at the expense of social insurance as feared by some representatives of social insurance institutions. Only about 8% of all adult patients implanted in Würzburg wanted a second implant being aware of the benefits and individual risks.

Considering the financial situation that might lead to only 50% of future patients receiving an implant if bilateral implantation became standard procedure, Laszig *et al*.[13] asked if bilateral cochlear implantation is ethically justifiable. There are two aspects to be considered: on the one hand, budget restrictions allow a certain number of patients to receive two implants or double that number to receive one implant; on the other hand, in the light of scientific evidence, children cannot be denied development of the second auditory pathway and the benefits of binaural hearing that is necessary in so many every-day situations.

There is also the question of whether it is justifiable to deny patients bilateral implantation for financial reasons after they have contributed to the social insurance system for many years and could now be kept fit for work by bilateral implantation (*i.e.* they will continue to pay taxes and contribute to social insurance). When discussing costs, economic and social aspects have to be considered. The problem here is that costs of implantation and subsequent financial relief affect different cost units.[10]

BILATERAL COCHLEAR IMPLANTATION TODAY

After very controversial discussions of bilateral cochlear implantation, the benefits and possible improvements, *i.e.* the basis for bilateral cochlear implantation, have been scientifically acknowledged. Switzerland was the first country to establish bilateral implantation as standard procedure. Scandinavia (Norway and Sweden) has also accepted bilateral implantation. At the 2nd Consensus Conference on Cochlear Implants in Valencia, a clear statement for bilateral cochlear implantation was made.[16] In Germany, costs for bilateral implantation in children and working adults are usually paid by social insurance.

CONCLUSIONS

Bilaterally implanted cochlear implant users using modern speech coding strategies experience clearly improved hearing and quality of life. Like people with normal hearing, they benefit from bilateral hearing because:

1. The cochlear implant systems work together and complement one another thus enabling binaural hearing.

2. The user has one ear 'closer' to the sound source on both sides.

3. The signal-to-noise ratio is better in the 'closer ear'.

4. Noise is less masking. Two cochlear implants enable a certain directional hearing and binaural cochlear implantation enables 'spatial hearing'.

5. A second cochlear implant can fill the 'gaps' of the first cochlear implant.

One patient, an English physicist, described his experiences very impressively after having received his second cochlear implant: 'I am back to the three-dimensional world'.

Key points for clinical practice

- Binaural hearing is essential for spatial hearing. The ability to localise a sound source depends on the interaural level, time difference and head shadow effect. It also allows estimation of the distance to a sound source.

- Bilateral cochlear implant users benefit from lasting improvement of speech understanding in quiet and in noise. It may restore spatial hearing, directional hearing and the separation of sound sources.

- Implanting simultaneously or sequentially is still a controversial topic among experts and cannot yet be fully answered.

- There is sufficient scientific evidence for bilateral cochlear implantation. Bilaterally implanted cochlear implant users clearly reveal improved hearing and quality of life.

References

1. Blauert J. *Räumliches Hören*. Stuttgart: S. Hirzel, 1974.
2. Hellbrück J. *Hören. Physiologie, Psychologie und Pathologie*. Göttingen: Hogrefe, 1993.
3. van Hoesel RJM, Tong YC, Hollow RD, Clark GM. Psychophysical and speech perception studies: a case report on a binaural cochlear implant subject. *J Acoust Soc Am* 1993; **94**: 3178–3189.
4. Wilson BS. pers. Mitteilung, Wullstein Symposium 2001, Würzburg.
5. Müller J. Ergebnisse der Bilateralen Cochlear Implant Versorgung. *Eur Arch Otorhinolaryngol* 1998; **255**: 38.
6. Müller J. Angemeldete Diskussionsbemerkung. Dt HNO-Kongress, Aachen 1999.
7. Leake PA, Hradek GT, Snyder RL. Chronic electrical stimulation by a cochlear implant promotes survival of spiral ganglion neurons after neonatal deafness. *J Comp Neurol* 1999; **412**: 543–562.
8. Müller J, Schön F, Helms J. Speech understanding in quiet and noise in bilateral users of the MED-EL COMBI 40/40+ cochlear implant system. *Ear Hear* 2002; **23**: 198–206.
9. Kühn-Inacker H, Shehata-Dieler W, Müller J, Helms J. Bilateral cochlear implants: a way to optimize auditory perception abilities in deaf children? *J Pediatr Otorhinolaryngol* 2004; **68**: 1257–1266.
10. Nopp P, Schleich P, D'Haese P. Sound localization in bilateral users of MED-EL COMBI 40/40+ cochlear implants. *Ear Hear* 2004; **25**: 205–214.
11. Schön F, Müller J, Helms J. Speech reception thresholds obtained in a symmetrical four-loudspeaker arrangement from bilateral users of MED-EL cochlear implants. *Otol Neurotol* 2002; **23**: 710–714.

12. Helms J, Muller J, Schon F, Brill S. Cochlea implantation: Ergebnisse und Kosten, eine Ubersicht. *Laryngorhinootologie* 2003; **82**: 821–825.

13. Laszig R, Aschendorff A, Schipper J, Klenzner T. Aktuelle Entwicklung zum Kochleaimplantat. *HNO* 2004; **52**: 357–362.

14. Bauer PW, Sharma A, Martin K, Dorman M. Central auditory development in children with bilateral cochlear implants. *Arch Otolaryngol Head Neck Surg* 2006; **132**: 1133–1136.

15. Sharma A, Dorman M-F, Kral AT. The influence of a sensitive period on central auditory development in children with unilateral and bilateral cochlear implants. *Hear Res* 2005; **203**: 134–143.

16. Offeciers E, Morera C, Muller J, Huarte A. Shallop J. Cavalle L. International consensus on bilateral cochlear implants and bimodal stimulation. *Acta Otolaryngol* 2005; **125**: 918–919.

17. Senn P, Kompis M, Vischer M, Haeusler R. Minimum audible angle, just noticeable interaural differences and speech intelligibility with bilateral cochlear implants using clinical speech processors. *Audiol Neurootol* 2005; **10**: 342–352.

18. Litovsky RY, Johnstone PM, Godar S et al. Bilateral cochlear implants in children: localization acuity measured with minimum audible angle. *Ear Hear* 2006; **27**: 43–59.

19. Litovsky RY, Parkinson A, Arcaroli J *et al*. Bilateral cochlear implants in adults and children. *Arch Otolaryngol Head Neck Surg* 2004; **130**: 648–655.

20. Nopp P, Schleich P, D'Haese P. Sound localization in bilateral users of MED-EL COMBI 40/40+ cochlear implants. *Ear Hear* 2004; **25**: 205–214.

21. Laszig R, Aschendorff A, Stecker M *et al*. Benefits of bilateral electrical stimulation with the nucleus cochlear implant in adults: 6-month postoperative results. *Otol Neurotol* 2004; **25**: 958–968.

22. Müller J. Wiederherstellende Verfahren bei gestörtem Hören: Die apparative Versorgung der Schwerhörigkeit: Cochlea Implantate und Hirnstammimplantate. Entwicklungen der letzten 10 Jahre. *Laryngorhinootologie* 2005; **84 (Suppl 1)**: 60–69.

23. Schoen F, Mueller J, Helms J, Nopp P. Sound localization and sensitivity to interaural cues in bilateral users of the Med-El Combi 40/40+ cochlear implant system. *Otol Neurotol* 2005; **26**: 429–437.

24. Schön F, Müller J, Helms J. Speech reception thresholds obtained in a symmetrical four-loudspeaker arrangement from bilateral users of MED-EL cochlear implants. *Otol Neurotol* 2002; **23**: 710–714.

25. Winkler F, Schön F, Peklo L, Müller J, Feinen C-h, Helms J. Wurzburger Fragebogen zur Horqualitat bei CI-Kindern (WH-CIK). Wurzburg questionnaire for assessing the quality of hearing in CI-children (WH-CIK). *Laryngorhinootologie* 2002; **81**: 211–216.

David A. Moffat Tim Price

5

Squamous cell carcinoma of the temporal bone: current evidence for radiotherapy alone and surgery with postoperative radiotherapy

Squamous cell carcinoma (SCC) of the temporal bone is a rare, highly malignant, aggressive disease in an extremely difficult anatomical site and has traditionally had a very poor prognosis. The prevalence of squamous carcinoma of the external auditory canal, middle ear and mastoid is said to be 1–6 per million of the population.[1] Its rarity has hampered the development of an evidence base for the most effective method of treatment as few surgeons or institutions have very much experience of this condition. The reliability of radiological evaluation of the extent of tumour invasion, the surgical options and extent of surgery and the efficacy of radiotherapy are still controversial. This chapter reviews the current evidence based on the recent literature and concentrates on squamous carcinoma of the temporal bone but excludes the rarer tumours that affect this site.

AETIOLOGY

Many factors have been implicated in the causation of SCC of the temporal bone. Like any SCC of the skin, UV light has been proposed as a causative agent. Although this is well documented with regards to the pinna, there is no evidence base for this in relation to the external auditory canal or those arising in the middle ear cleft.

Many textbooks and papers implicate chronic suppurative otitis media (CSOM) as an aetiological factor but there is no evidence base for this statement. However, it is purported that approximately 50% of patients

David A. Moffat BSc MA FRCS (for correspondence)
Consultant in Otoneurological and Skull Base Surgery, Box 48, Addenbrooke's Hospital, Hills Road, Cambridge CB1 1QQ, UK
E-mail: dam26@cam.ac.uk

Tim Price BSc DLO FRCS (ORL HNS)
Consultant ENT Surgeon, Dorset County Hospital, Dorchester, UK

presenting with squamous cell carcinoma of the temporal bone have had a preceding period of chronic suppurative otitis media.[2]

Radiation-associated tumours are well described in the literature. These arise following initial radiotherapy for lesions in close anatomical proximity,

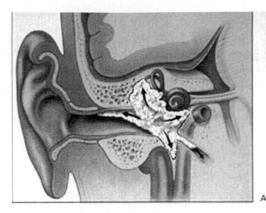

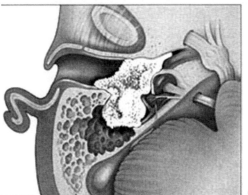

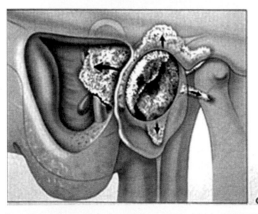

Fig. 1 (A) Coronal section of a very advanced temporal bone SCC illustrating the lines of spread within the temporal bone superiorly, medially and laterally. (B) Axial view of the lesion demonstrating spread anteriorly, posteriorly, medially and laterally. (C) Parasagittal view showing anterior, posterior, superior and inferior spread. (From *Tumors of the ear and temporal bone*. Jackler and Driscoll. (eds) New York: Lippincott Williams and Wilkins, 2000, Figure 18.3 'Squamous cell carcinoma', Chapter 5, page 71. Reproduced with kind permission of the editors.)

Table 1 Frequency of presenting symptoms

	Nyrop & Grontved[8]	Moffat et al.[2,9]	Gillespie et al.[10]	Moody et al.[22]
Otorrhoea	45%	69%	73%	75%
Otalgia	35%	64%	53%	81%
Hearing loss	25%		33%	22%
Facial palsy		17%	13%	25%

for example, in the treatment of nasopharyngeal carcinoma.[3] Lustig et al.[4] report a latency time with a mean of 12.9 years post-treatment and Goh et al.[5] 15 years.

Many other aetiological factors have been reported, but dismissed, such as chlorinated disinfectants.[6]

EPIDEMIOLOGY

SCC has previously been reported to have a higher incidence in women[7] but, more recently, the incidence would appear to be equal in men and women.[8,9]

PEAK INCIDENCE

SCC of the temporal bone occurs most commonly in the fifth and sixth decade of life.[8–10]

CLINICAL SYMPTOMS

These relate to the primary anatomical site of origin of the tumour and the direction of spread of disease (Fig. 1). Many presenting symptoms are not specific to the disease and are seen in CSOM but severe pain, blood-stained discharge from the ear and facial palsy should arouse suspicion. Table 1 lists the most frequently described symptoms.

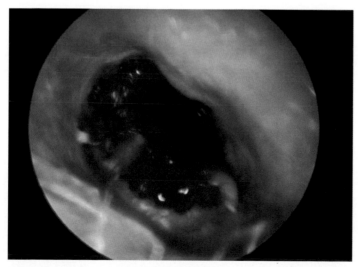

Fig. 2 Otoscopic view of a squamous carcinoma of the external auditory canal showing the characteristic exophytic friable bleeding mass.

CLINICAL SIGNS

The signs may also be non-specific and mimic inflammatory disease. An exophytic mass that bleeds when touched is the most diagnostic feature (Fig. 2).

Polypoid tissue with fissures in the ear canal, cranial nerve palsies and pre- and postauricular masses (which may be ulcerated) are other common presentations.

PATTERNS OF SPREAD

The lymphatic supply of the ear canal is not well developed; therefore, lymphatic spread to local nodes is relatively uncommon and late in the disease process. The incidence is between 10–23% of patients.[11]

SCC has a strong predisposition for perineural spread. As a result of the anatomical position of the facial nerve within the temporal bone, it is commonly involved (17–25%).[12] Haematogenous spread from the temporal bone to distant sites is very rare and mortality is most often due to locoregional disease recurrence.[9]

MANAGEMENT

DIAGNOSIS

Histological confirmation following biopsy is the gold standard of diagnosis (Fig. 3). There is inevitably a degree of secondary infection and oedema of the surface of these lesions within the ear canal; therefore, biopsies must be deep and not just include superficial tissue or the underlying carcinoma will be missed. This may necessitate a deep biopsy under a general anaesthetic.

CT-guided fine needle biopsy is possible but rarely required even for deeper lesions in the middle ear cleft since they can usually be seen under the microscope.[13]

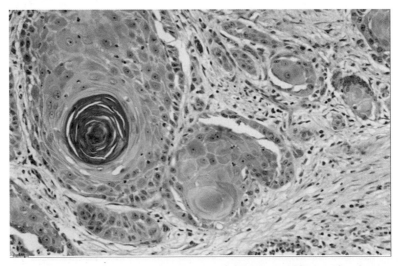

Fig. 3 Histopathology of squamous carcinoma of the temporal bone. The characteristic epithelial whorl with layers of keratin in the centre can be clearly seen.

Of tumours of the temporal bone, 80% are squamous cell carcinomas but the differential diagnosis includes basal cell carcinoma (BCC), adenocarcinoma, chondrosarcoma, melanoma, Ewing's tumour, Langerhans' histiocytosis X, fibroxanthoma, verrucous carcinoma and metastatic disease.[11] Recently, pseudo-epitheliomatous hyperplasia has been included in the differential.[14]

INVESTIGATIONS

Imaging

A combination of CT scan and magnetic resonance imaging (MRI) are required for accurate pre-operative assessment as they are complimentary techniques in lesions of the skull base. CT scans are the modality of choice for the detection of bony erosion, which may be the only sign of underlying sinister pathology (Fig. 4). MRI scans are necessary to elucidate the extent of soft tissue involvement, perineural spread and dural enhancement (Fig. 5).

In 1984, Sataloff et al.[15] proposed the total en bloc resection of the temporal bone and carotid artery for malignant tumours of the temporal bone. In these cases, arteriography was necessary to provide pre-operative information about the potential cross flow from the circle of Willis and allowed a balloon occlusion test to be performed – a potentially risky procedure. Graham et al.[16] demonstrated that the morbidity and mortality in patients following carotid sacrifice was so great that it was not justified. Thus, most surgeons would hope

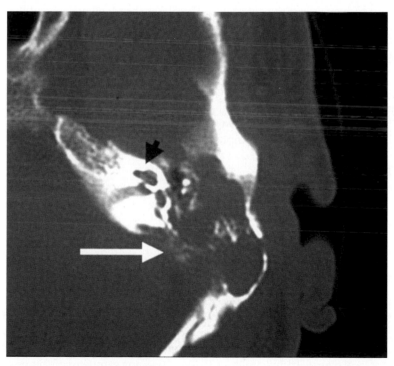

Fig. 4 Axial CT scan with bony windows of left temporal bone showing massive irregular erosion of the lateral temporal bone. The black arrow indicates that the cochlea and petrous apex are intact. The white arrow demonstrated extensive erosion of the posterior face of the temporal bone.

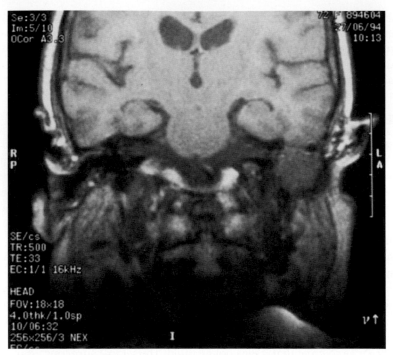

Fig. 5 Coronal MRI T1-weighted image with gadolinium DTPA enhancement showing a large squamous carcinoma of the left temporal bone demonstrating dural enhancement due to tumour involvement of the adjacent dura and temporal lobe of the brain.

not to sacrifice the internal carotid artery but, if the imaging suggests possible carotid involvement, then cross-flow studies are necessary.[9,10]

A chest X-ray is necessary as part of the staging of disease; if systemic disease is suspected, a radionucleotide or PET scan confirms or excludes systemic spread before aggressive surgical management is considered. Extended temporal bone resection can, however, be performed as a palliative procedure in view of the unacceptable demise of the untreated patient.

Audiology

Pre-operative audiometric assessment of the contralateral ear is mandatory.

STAGING

The lack of a universally accepted staging system has hampered the comparison of studies between institutions, making it difficult to compare results and define the best form of treatment for this disease.

In 1980, Goodwin and Jesse[17] described a 3-stage system derived from involvement of the external auditory canal, tympanic membrane, or extension to the middle ear and beyond. In 1985, Stell and McCormick[18] designed a staging system based on the anatomical origin of tumour (external auditory canal or middle ear) and the extent of local spread. In this system, a T3 lesion was any extratemporal bone spread.

Clark et al.[19] later split extratemporal T3 lesions into those that had a more favourable outcome (parotid, temporomandibular joint and skin involvement) and those with poorer outcomes (involvement of the dura and skull base).

Table 2 Hirsch's modified Pittsburgh Staging System

T1	Tumour limited to the EAC without bony erosion or evidence of soft tissue extension
T2	Tumour with limited EAC erosion (not full thickness) or radiological findings consistent with limited (< 0.05 cm) soft tissue involvement
T3	Tumour eroding the osseous EAC (full thickness) with limited (< 0.05 cm) soft tissue involvement of middle ear and/or mastoid, or causing facial paralysis at presentation
T4	Tumour eroding the cochlear, petrous apex, medial wall of middle ear, carotid canal, jugular foramen, or dura, or with extensive (> 0.05 cm) soft tissue involvement
N status	Lymph node involvement is a poor prognostic sign and places the patient in an advanced stage (*i.e.* T1N1 [stage III] and T2–4N1 [Stage IV])
M status	M1 disease is stage IV and is considered a very poor prognostic sign

Arriaga *et al.*[20] devised a system that conformed to the American Joint Cancer Committee's TNM classification. This system is known as the University of Pittsburgh Staging System. It provides a prediction of outcome based on the stage of the disease. A number of authors have found good correlation between the stage of disease and curative outcome with this system.[8,9,21,22]

Hirsch[12] modified the staging system to upgrade the importance of facial nerve involvement (Table 2). He believes that facial nerve involvement is a defining feature of a T3 carcinoma. For the facial nerve to be clinically involved, the tumour must have invaded the medial wall of the middle ear cavity or extended beyond the boundaries of the mastoid into the infratemporal space to invade the nerve at the stylomastoid foramen. However, Moffat *et al.*[9] did not find facial nerve involvement to be a significant prognostic indicator. The Pittsburgh Staging System is now the most commonly used system.[1]

TREATMENT

RADIOTHERAPY

Radiotherapy as the sole treatment modality is rare.[1] In the early years because of poor surgical outcomes in terms of patient morbidity and poor survival rates, radiotherapy was used as the primary treatment to attempt a cure. The published survival rates for all tumours including early T1 and T2 lesions varied from 23–42%. However, an unspecified number of these patients underwent various forms of radical mastoidectomy and postoperative radiotherapy.[23–26]

Very early (T1) cancers of the pinna and external ear canal have had good control rates with radiotherapy alone but many authors have shown increased survival rates for more advanced tumours with combined surgery and radiotherapy as opposed to either of these modalities used on their own.[22,25–28].

Usually, 60–70 Gy is given as a total dose to both the primary site and the neck. Those patients who have previously undergone radiotherapy prior to

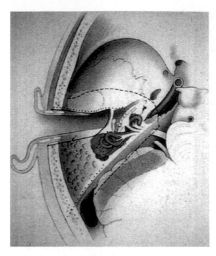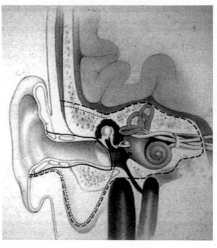

Fig. 6 The concept of *en bloc* resection of the temporal bone is illustrated in the axial (left) and coronal planes (right). Sleeve resection of the external auditory canal (solid line) is rarely indicated for small, lesions of the EAC. Lateral temporal bone resection (dotted line) is indicated for most cancers limited to the EAC. Total temporal bone resection (dashed line) is indicated for advanced temporal bone cancer and is performed by a combination of en bloc and piecemeal resection techniques, rather than neatly as shown in this diagram. (Reproduced from: Robert K. Jackler MD. *Atlas of Neuro-otology and Skull Base Surgery*. St Louis, Mosby, 1996 with kind permission of the editor.)

surgical resection can receive further postoperative radiotherapy because the irradiated tissues can be widely excised and the flap reconstruction provides sufficient new blood supply to enable patients to tolerate a second dose.[9]

Complications include osteoradionecrosis of the temporal bone and facial weakness.

SURGERY

Many publications advocate surgery alone for early T1 tumours followed by postoperative radiotherapy for those with a positive surgical margin. For all T2–4 tumours, surgery followed by adjuvant radiotherapy is the treatment of choice. All skull base surgeons and neuro-otologists would accept this concept of management but the exact type or extent of the surgery involved is still a matter for heated debate.

Surgery for T1 and T2 lesions

For very early T1 tumours, a 'sleeve resection' (the removal of a circumferential 'sleeve' of ear canal skin with the enclosed tumour) may be adequate (Fig. 6). However, as these tumours are notoriously aggressive and difficult to diagnose early, this operation is only going to be sufficient in a small minority of cases.

Most skull base surgeons would recommend a lateral temporal bone resection (LTBR) for T1 and T2 lesions (Fig. 6). This involves removal of the entire pinna with a surrounding oval of skin and an *en bloc* resection of the temporal bone lateral to the stapes, facial nerve and otic capsule.[1] In some instances where there is healthy meatal skin laterally in the external canal and meatus, it may be possible to conserve the helix of the pinna which is useful for those patients who wear glasses.

Treasure[29] reported two cases of external auditory canal carcinoma presenting with temporomandibular joint (TMJ) pain and invasion. In view of the close proximity of the TMJ to the external auditory canal and middle ear, Moffat et al.[9] recommended resection of the head of the mandible and TMJ. Primarily this is because the anterior wall of the ear canal is thin and erosion of the bone is common and may be difficult to detect on CT scanning. Excision of the TMJ ensures an adequate anterior resection margin.[9]

Moffat et al.[9] also recommended a superficial parotidectomy for T1 and T2 lesions in order to remove the first echelon nodes draining the external canal. This technique is more radical than that proposed by many other authors. They propose doing a radical mastoidectomy and postoperative radiotherapy and have similar survival rates to LTBR.[1] Nyrop and Grontved[8] stated that local external auditory canal resection aided by frozen section is a reasonable approach for stage I and II disease and reported a survival rate of 92%.

However, a radical mastoidectomy is an operation designed for chronic inflammatory disease. It involves piecemeal removal of the temporal bone and does not provide a tumour margin. This goes against all oncological surgical principles; as the resultant defect is very similar to that left by a LTBR, it would appear that an LTBR is a better oncological procedure. Survival rates of 100% for T2 tumours as reported by Moffat et al.[9] would support this view.

Surgery for T3 and T4 disease

Most skull base surgeons would agree that stage III and IV tumours require more extensive surgery, followed by postoperative radiotherapy, in order to effect a cure. This is supported by a meta-analysis performed by Prasad and Janecka,[30] which showed an obvious decrease in survival rates with lesser operations for SCC of the middle ear.

Exactly how the surgery is carried out is still a matter for debate. The common approach has been to perform a LTBR and then to remove the rest of the tumour in a piecemeal fashion.[1] However, for the same reasons given above, an *en bloc* resection would seem more appropriate despite the difficulty of achieving this in view of the pyramidal shape of the temporal bone. This is achieved by performing a subtotal temporal bone resection (STBR) or a total temporal bone resection (TTBR), which is also know as an extended temporal bone resection (Fig. 6).

Both Moffat et al.[2] and Nyrop and Grontved[8] agree that the extended temporal bone resection is appropriate for stage III and IV disease. Extended temporal bone resection for T3 and T4 lesions has been described in detail by Moffat et al.[2] The resection includes the entire petrous temporal bone lateral to the carotid artery including sacrificing the facial nerve, the parotid gland, the mandible and soft tissue of the infratemporal fossa. These are removed in one specimen alone with 3 cm of temporal bone posterior to the sigmoid sinus. If the carotid artery appears involved, Moffat et al.[2] recommend peeling the tumour off the adventitia of the arterial wall and it is rarely so deeply involved that sacrifice becomes necessary.

The apex of the temporal bone is the only component removed as a separate specimen.

Moffat *et al.*[9] found involvement of the local lymph nodes draining the temporal bone was a poor prognostic indicator; therefore, management of the neck is an integral part of disease treatment. Nakagawa *et al.*[31] also found that node stage was the factor most associated with patient survival.

Clinically, negative neck disease is treated with a supra-omohyoid neck dissection. This allows staging of the disease for postoperative radiotherapy; it also allows control of the great vessels of the neck and access to the skull base to be obtained. Exposed vessels are then preserved for anastomosis with the free flap repair.[11]

Resection of involved dura and brain is carried out when the main specimen has been removed. Although invasion of these structures, can be delineated by MRI scanning with gadolinium DTPA enhancement, intra-operative assessment is definitive. Abnormal temporal lobe is removed macroscopically with a rim of normal brain tissue. The dural margins are sent for frozen section to ensure histological clearance of dura. This allows the minimal amount of dura to be resected. This is important medially as it preserves as much dura as possible to allow a watertight fascial seal to be created.[11]

RECONSTRUCTION

A variety of reconstructive techniques can be employed in the head and neck in a graduated sequence. Following temporal bone resection, the reconstruction requires muscle bulk and skin coverage. The two most common types of reconstructive techniques in use are: (i) a pedicled myocutaneous flap; and (ii) a free tissue transfer. The choice of flap is dependent on patient factors, size of surgical defect, the surgical skills and experience of the reconstructive unit and postoperative nursing care.[11]

Nowadays, the most common free flap repair is lateral upper thigh in males (Fig. 7) and the upper outer arm in females. The upper outer arm free flap

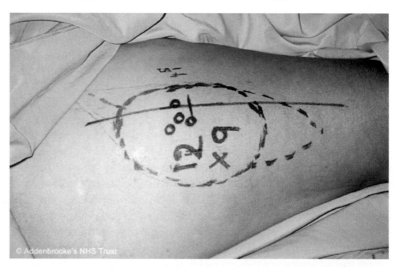

Fig. 7 Right lateral upper thigh free flap marked out pre-operatively. This flap is used more commonly in male patients because there is not enough subcutaneous tissue in the arm to allow the direct closure of upper outer arm flaps unlike female patients where this is usually possible.

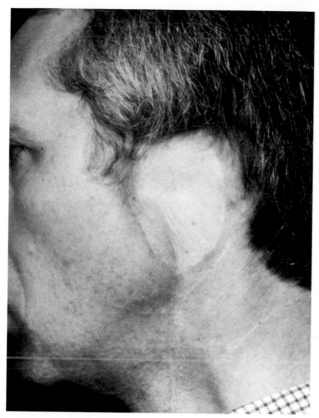

Fig. 8 The final cosmetic appearance of a free flap based on the anterior cubital artery in the arm (modified Chinese flap). This was performed to reconstruct the defect after an extended temporal bone resection for squamous cell carcinoma with dural and temporal lobe involvement. The patient is alive and well 12 years later.

incision can be closed primarily without skin grafting in view of the amount of subcutaneous tissue in females. In males, where the subcutaneous tissue is less and precludes direct closure, the upper outer thigh is preferred. The cosmetic result of free flap reconstruction following extended temporal bone resection is very acceptable (Fig. 8).

COMPLICATIONS

The facial nerve is sacrificed in total temporal bone resection for T3 and T4 tumours. Rehabilitation focuses on corneal protection. An upper eyelid weight insertion or inner or outer canthoplasties may be necessary, particularly if there is marked ectropion present. Static procedures for facial palsy will improve the appearance of the face at rest but are only considered once the reconstructive flap has a well-established blood supply.

Lower cranial nerve palsies (glossopharyngeal [IX], vagal [X], and accessory [XI]) are inevitable in some cases when directly involved by the tumour or when the resection margin dictates a reasonable clearance. If they occur, they are compounded by poor facial nerve function and resection of the head of the mandible.[11]

Rehabilitation to improve both speech and airway protection involves both vocal cord medialization procedures (collagen injection or thyroplasty) and percutaneous gastrostomy insertion for feeding purposes may be necessary, particularly in the elderly.

CSF leak is a potential complication of any skull base procedure when the dura is breached. Prevention occurs with good watertight fascial closure and postoperative lumbar drain insertion.[11]

PROGNOSIS

In most studies, the cure rate is high when the disease remains lateral to the tympanic membrane (T1 and T2 carcinomas) and ranges from 80–100%.[9,10,22] As previously mentioned, the main controversy revolves around whether a larger operation gives better results for advanced disease. It is difficult to compare series as the authors have used different staging systems, have not separated out their results for the various stages of disease, and the numbers of patients in each group are generally too small to achieve statistical significance. However, the meta-analysis of Prasads and Janecka[30] would tend to support the notion that the more radical the surgery, the better the patient outcome.

The survival rates for T3 and T4 tumours treated with radical mastoidectomy and postoperative radiotherapy range from 53–69%.[26,32,33] However, the survival rates for T4 tumours are poor at around 20%.[26]

Initially, Nyrop and Grontved[8] advocated performing a piecemeal resection of tumours but finally reached the conclusion that *en bloc* resection is more likely to offer a curative result. Moffat *et al.*[9] and Moody *et al.*[22] both recommend an *en bloc* resection; Moody *et al.*[22] proposed that a prospective protocol is developed so that each skull base unit follow a progression of treatment that is specific for each stage of the disease based on a consistent staging system. They suggest that, for early lesions, a modified temporal bone resection or a lateral temporal bone resection (LTBR) is performed. For more advanced lesions, a subtotal temporal bone resection (STBR) or a total temporal bone resection (TTBR) should be the treatment of choice.

Moffat *et al.*[2] adopted a more radical approach than this and stated that the minimal procedure for disease lateral to the tympanic membrane should be a LTBR and superficial parotidectomy. For T3 and T4 disease, an extended temporal bone resection and total parotidectomy with facial nerve sacrifice offers the greatest chance of cure.

Following this surgical technique, Moffat *et al.*[9] have achieved survival rates of 100% for T3N0 tumours and 50% overall for all T3 stage disease and 38% for T4 disease (Table 3).

Table 3 Survival related to stage of TNM classification (*n* = 37)

Stage	TNM	Number	TNM survival	Stage survival	T stage	T stage survival
Stage II	T2N0M0	2	100%	100%	T2	100%
Stage III	T3N0M0	3	100%	100%	T3	50%
Stage IV	T3N1N0	3	0%			50%
	T4N1M0	23	47.8%	34.3%	T4	38%
	T4N1M0	6	0%			

PROGNOSTIC FACTORS

NODAL DISEASE

Moffat et al.[9] reported that 23% of patients had nodal disease at presentation. This was the most significant prognostic indicator, as survival in this group at 2 years was 0%. Death was always due to local recurrence and hence these authors believe that nodal disease is a good indicator of aggressive disease. Nakagawa et al.[31] have recently concurred with this finding.

HISTOLOGY

Survival rate can be directly correlated with the degree of differentiation of the tumour.[9,11] Well differentiated tumours appear to have been better controlled with aggressive therapy than poorly differentiated tumours which had much reduced chances of disease control despite aggressive therapy.[9,34]

HISTOLOGICAL POSITIVE MARGINS

Positive histological margins at the time of resection, not surprisingly, are a poor prognostic indicator in this locally aggressive disease. Death in these patients is usually within 12 months.

DURAL AND CEREBRAL INVOLVEMENT

Dural involvement has been stated to be a bad prognostic indicator.[22,31] However, in the series of Moffat and colleagues, dural involvement alone was not a significant prognostic indicator. Brain involvement is usually associated with a very poor outcome. However, one patient remains alive, 12 years after an extended temporal bone resection and a partial temporal lobe resection.[9,11]

CAROTID INVASION

Invasion of the carotid artery signifies extensive disease progression and has a poor outcome.[9,10,34] Involvement of the carotid is not as common as imagined. The tumour is more likely to spread superiorly to the middle fossa dura, anteriorly into the temporomandibular joint or inferiorly to the jugular bulb rather than medially to the intrapetrous carotid. Even if the carotid is involved, it is usually possible to peel the tumour off the adventitia of the artery. Moody et al.[22] successfully resected the carotid in one patient who is still alive, but no comment was made with regards to neurological status in this case.

DE NOVO SURGERY VERSUS SALVAGE SURGERY

Moffat et al.[9] analysed their patients according to previous management. If they had undergone any treatment at another institution, then further treatment was deemed as salvage. Those patients with no previous treatment were defined as de novo cases. Although the numbers were too small to make any statistical analysis, the trend showed poorer outcomes for the salvage patients with a comparable stage of disease. This would support the concept that the first treatment protocol offers the greatest chance of cure and supports the argument for these patients to be referred early to those few centres who have the experience to deal with these cases (Table 4).

Table 4 *De novo* versus salvage surgery (survival in T4N0 group; *n* = 23)

	De novo surgery	Salvage surgery
T4N0	11	12
Alive	7	4
Dead	4	8
	63%	33%

RADIATION-ASSOCIATED TUMOUR

In the series of Lim *et al.*,[3] the trend was for radiation-associated tumour to have a poorer prognosis. The 1-year cumulative recurrence rate for this group was 100%.

THE FUTURE

Chemotherapy has previously been thought to be of little benefit but Knegt *et al.*[35] described a report of tumour debulking followed by repeated application of 5-fluorouracil. The overall 5-year survival rate was 74% in a study where 65% of the lesions were T1 and T2.

In 2006, Nakagawa *et al.*[31] described using pre-operative chemoradiotherapy for advanced disease. They were able to down-stage the disease before surgery and, in 50% of T3 and T4 tumours, no tumour was found in the surgically resected specimen.[31] The numbers of patients were very small; therefore, caution should be used when analysing these results but chemoradiotherapy may be very useful in the future particularly when dealing with well and moderately differentiated tumours.

Key points for clinical practice

- Squamous cell carcinoma of the external auditory canal and temporal bone is a rare tumour.

- Many presenting symptoms are not specific to the disease and are seen in chronic suppurative otitis media but severe pain, blood stained discharge from the ear and facial palsy should arouse suspicion.

- Biopsies must be deep and not just include superficial tissue or the underlying carcinoma will be missed.

- A combination of computed tomography and magnetic resonance imaging are required for accurate pre-operative assessment of the extent of bony erosion and soft tissue involvement.

- The University of Pittsburgh Staging System is now the most commonly used classification system.

- Radiotherapy as the sole treatment modality is now rare, particularly for T3 and T4 tumours.

- Radical *en bloc* extended temporal bone resection followed by post-operative radiotherapy offers the best chance for T3 and T4 lesions.

References

1. Barrs DM. Temporal bone carcinoma. *Otolaryngol Clin North Am* 2001; **34**: 1197–1218.
2. Moffat DA, Grey P, Ballagh RH, Hardy DG. Extended temporal bone resection for squamous cell carcinoma. *Otolaryngol Head Neck Surg* 1997; **116**: 617–623.
3. Lim LH, Goh YH, Chan M, Chong VF, Low WK. Malignancy of the temporal bone and external auditory canal. *Otolaryngol Head Neck Surg* 2000; **122**: 882–886.
4. Lustig LR, Jackler RK, Lanser MJ. Radiation-induced tumours of the temporal bone. *Am J Otol* 1997; **18**: 230–235.
5. Goh YH, Chong VF, Low WK. Temporal bone tumours in patients irradiated for nasopharyngeal neoplasm. *J Laryngol Otol* 1999; **113**: 222–228.
6. Monem SA, Moffat DA, Frampton, MC. Carcinoma of the ear: a case report of a possible association with chlorinated disinfectants. *J Laryngol Otol* 1999; **13**: 1004–1007.
7. Morton RP, Stell PH, Derrick PPO. Epidemiology of cancer of the middle ear cleft. *Cancer* 1984; **53**: 1612–1617.
8. Nyrop M, Grontved A. Cancer of the external auditory canal. *Arch Otolaryngol Head Neck Surg* 2002; **128**: 834–837.
9. Moffat DA, Wagstaff SA, Hardy DG. The outcome of radical surgery and post-operative radiotherapy for squamous carcinoma of the temporal bone. *Laryngoscope* 2005; **115**: 341 347.
10. Gillespie MB, Francis HW, Chee N, Eisele DW. Squamous cell carcinoma of the temporal bone: a radiographic-pathologic correlation. *Arch Otolaryngol Head Neck Surg* 2001; **127**: 803–807.
11. Moffat DA, Wagstaff SA. Squamous cell carcinoma of the temporal bone. *Curr Opin Otolaryngol Head Neck Surg* 2003; **11**: 107 111.
12. Hirsch BE. Staging system revision. *Arch Otolaryngol Head Neck Surg* 2002; **128**: 93–94.
13. Zaharopoulos P. Carcinoma of the temporal bone, base of the skull: diagnosis by needle aspiration cytology. *Diagn Cytopathol* 2001; **24**: 356–360.
14. Gacek MR, Gacek RR, Gantz B, McKenna M, Goodman M. Pseudoepitheliomatous hyperplasia versus squamous cell carcinoma of the external auditory canal. *Auris Nasus Larynx* 2001; **28**: 169–172.
15. Sataloff RT, Myers DL, Lowry LD et al. Total temporal bone resection for squamous cell carcinoma. *Otolaryngol Head Neck Surg* 1987; **96**: 5–14.
16. Graham MD, Sataloff RT, Wolf GT et al. Total *en bloc* resection of the temporal bone and carotid artery for malignant tumours of the ear and temporal bone. *Laryngoscope* 1984; **94**: 528–533.
17. Goodwin WJ, Jesse R. Malignant neoplasms of the EAC and temporal bone. *Arch Otolaryngol* 1980; **106**: 675–679.
18. Stell PM, McCormick MS. Carcinoma of the external auditory meatus and middle ear. Prognostic factors and suggested staging system. *J Laryngol Otol* 1985; **99**: 847–850.
19. Clark LJ, Narula AA, Morgan DA et al. Squamous carcinoma of the temporal bone: a revised staging. *J Laryngol Otol* 1991; **105**: 346 348.
20. Arriaga M, Curtin H, Takahashi H, Hirsch BE, Kamerer DB. Staging proposal for external auditory meatus carcinoma based on preoperative clinical examination and computed tomography findings. *Ann Otol Rhinol Laryngol* 1990; **99**: 714–721.
21. Austin JR, Stewart KL, Fawzi N. Therapeutic prognosis based on a proposed staging system. *Arch Otolaryngol Head Neck Surg* 1994; **120**: 1228–1232.
22. Moody SA, Hirsch BE, Myers EN. Squamous cell carcinoma of the external auditory canal: an evaluation of a staging system. *Am J Otol* 2000; **21**: 582–588.
23. Boland J, Paterson R. Cancer of the middle ear and external auditory meatus. *J Laryngol Otol* 1955; **69**: 468–478.
24. Holmes KS. Carcinoma of the middle ear. *Clin Radiol* 1965; **16**: 400–404.
25. Arthur K. Radiotherapy in carcinoma of the middle ear and auditory canal. *J Laryngol Otol* 1976; **90**: 753–762.
26. Birzgalis AR, Keith AO, Farrington WT. Radiotherapy in the treatment of middle ear and mastoid carcinoma. *Clin Otolaryngol* 1992; **17**: 113–116.
27. Korzeniowski S, Pszon J. The results of radiotherapy of cancer of the middle ear. *Int J Radiat Oncol Biol Phys* 1990; **18**: 631–633.
28. Hahn SS, Kim JA, Goodchild N. Carcinoma of the middle ear and EAC. *Int J Radiat*

Oncol Biol Phys 1983; **9**: 1003–1007.

29. Treasure T. External auditory canal carcinoma involving the temporomandibular joint: two cases presenting as temporomandibular disorders. *J Oral Maxillofac Surg* 2002; **60**: 465–469.

30. Prasad S, Janecka IP. Efficacy of surgical treatments for squamous cell carcinoma of the temporal bone: a literature review. *Otolaryngol Head Neck Surg* 1994; **110**: 270–280.

31. Nakagawa T, Kumamoto Y, Natori Y *et al.* Squamous cell carcinoma of the external auditory canal and middle ear: an operation combined with preoperative chemoradiotherapy and a free surgical margin. *Otol Neurotol* 2006; **27**: 242–249.

32. Chao CK, Sheen TS, Shau WY *et al.* Treatment, outcomes and prognostic factors of ear canal. *J Formos Med Assoc* 1999; **98**: 314–318.

33. Liu FF, Keane TJ, Davidson J. Primary carcinoma involving the petrous temporal bone. *Head Neck* 1993; **15**: 39–43.

34. Shih L, Crabtree JA. Carcinoma of the external auditory canal: an update. *Laryngoscope* 1990; **100**: 1215–1218.

35. Knegt PP, Ah-See KW, Meeuwis CA, Van Der Velden LA, Kerrebijn JDF, De Boer MF. Squamous carcinoma of the external auditory canal: a different approach. *Clin Otolaryngol* 2002; **27**: 183–187.

Holger Sudhoff Désirée Garten Sören Schreiber

6

Reflux and otitis media with effusion

DEFINITIONS

GER/GERD

Gastro-oesophageal reflux (GER) occurs when gastric contents pass through the lower oesophageal sphincter (LES) into the oesophagus. If GER causes symptoms or findings such as mucosal irritation or further damage, this is defined as gastro-oesophageal reflux disease (GERD).[1]

EER/EERD

From the oesophagus, the refluxate can emerge into the upper and lower airways, nose, nasopharynx, oral cavity and middle ear and this is referred as extra-oesophageal reflux (EER) which may also proceed to mucosal lesions called extra-oesophageal reflux disease (EERD). EER is increasingly recognized as a causative agent of different respiratory and otolaryngological disorders in adult and paediatric patients. Refluxed gastric content plays an important role in asthma,[2] chronic cough,[3] laryngitis,[3] vocal cord nodules,[4] recurrent croup,[4] subglottic stenosis,[3,4] globus,[3] laryngeal carcinoma[3] and pharyngitis. EER may also be the underlying cause of infantile apnoea.[4] In addition, increasing evidence shows that EER is also involved in the

Holger Sudhoff MD PhD (for correspondence)
Professor, Chairman and Medical Director, Department of Otorhinolaryngology, Head and Neck Surgery, Bielefeld Academic Teaching Hospital, Teutoburger Strasse 50, 33604 Bielefeld, Germany
E-mail: holger.sudhoff @ sk-bielefeld.de

Désirée Garten
Physician Scientist, Institut für Physiologie der Ruhr-Universität Bochum, Germany

Sören Schreiber MD PhD
Associate Professor, Institut für Physiologie der Ruhr-Universität Bochum, Germany

pathogenesis of sinusitis,[4] oropharyngeal dysphagia,[3] chronic rhinosinusitis,[4,5] adenoid hypertrophy,[6] laryngomalacia,[4] otalgia and forms of otitis, particularly otitis media with effusion.[4,7,8]

OTITIS MEDIA

Otitis media (OM), a common otorhinolaryngological disorder, is either presented as acute OM or otitis media with effusion (OME). The inflammation of the middle ear is diagnosed more than 5 million times per year in the US. Thus OM is, after simple respiratory infections, the second most common disease in childhood.

The highest prevalence of OM is observed during the first 2 years of life, but it is highly prevalent throughout preschool aged children. Acute OM shows a rapid symptom onset and marked otoscopic findings for inflammation.[9]

OTITIS MEDIA WITH EFFUSION

Otitis media with effusion (OME), defined as an asymptomatic middle-ear effusion persistent for at least 3 months without any signs or symptoms of active inflammation, is possibly associated with a 'plugged ear' feeling. In some cases, it occurs as the first manifestation of inflammatory processes in the middle ear or a sequela of a previous ear infection.

By the age of 3 years, 83% of all infants experience one or more episodes of otitis media with effusion.[10] Despite being a frequent cause for deafness in children in the developed world, the pathogenesis of OME is not completely understood.

Several aetiological factors have been reported including eustachian tube dysfunction, allergies, inflammatory mediators identified in the eustachian tube and the middle ear, viral and bacterial infections.[9,11] Additionally, recent research implicates an important role of EER in the multifactorial pathogenesis of this chronic inflammatory condition.

The purpose of this article is to discuss the role of extra-oesophageal reflux in OME. Hence, the aetiology of both disorders, the pathophysiological mechanism of interaction between GER and OME, the prevalence of EER in patients with OME and the success of antireflux treatment among OME patients will be discussed. Important features concerning diagnosis and therapy of EERD will be given.

AETIOLOGY OF GERD AND EERD

PREVALENCE OF GERD AND EERD

About 75 million (15–44%) of all American adults experience 'heartburn',[12] which characterizes GERD, one of the most common gastrointestinal disorders. Approximately 50% of these patients show symptoms of EER.[12] Among paediatric patients, GER is also common,[13] whereas the prevalence of GERD is unknown.[1] GERD is increasingly diagnosed in adults above the age of 40 years and has a higher prevalence in Western countries. Due to various symptoms, the prevalence of EERD in infants and children can only be estimated at 1.8–22%.[14]

MECHANISM UNDERLYING GER

Occurring in 70–100% of reflux episodes, transient lower oesophageal sphincter relaxations (TLESRs) are the main mechanism underlying GER. TLESRs are defined as prolonged relaxations of the lower oesophageal sphincter (LES) not associated with swallowing. Under resting conditions, the LES maintains an intraluminal pressure higher than the gastric fundus pressure, thereby preventing GER. During TLESR, the LES tone completely relaxes for 10–45 s. In contrast to TLESR, a low basal pressure of the LES underlies GER only in patients with a severe oesophagitis. Distension of the stomach normally caused by ingested food, triggers TLESR as the major stimulus without acting on the resting LES pressure.[15]

PATHOLOGICAL GER/EER

Acidic reflux is considered to be pathological if the oesophageal pH is lower than 4 for a given percentage of time (e.g. 4%) during a 24-h pH-metry.[16] During the first year of life, GER physiologically occurs in neonates and infants. Vomiting and regurgitation are regarded as the major symptoms of GER in the paediatric population. However, recurrent vomiting is common during the first months of life but than decreases progressively.

PHYSIOLOGICAL MECHANISMS PROTECTING THE OESOPHAGUS

The oesophagus is protected by frequent swallows that clear material, the buffering capacity of saliva squamous epithelium, and tonic contraction of the LES. Saliva produced at physiological rates neutralizes small amounts of intra-oesophageal acid within minutes and this ability to neutralize acid is mainly attributable to bicarbonate. Oesophageal acid clearance involves one or two peristaltic sequences, which leave a minimal volume of acid within the oesophagus. The remaining acid is neutralized by swallowed saliva.

PATHOGENESIS OF MUCOSAL INJURY

It is frequently observed that retrograde reflux consisting of hydrochloric acid, active pepsin, bile and pancreatic enzymes contribute to secondary disease processes. Experimental evidence has shown that acid alone is substantially less potent in causing injury than a combination of acid and the gastric protease pepsin. Particularly within the pH range 2.0–3.5, pepsin damages the oesophageal mucosa. Above pH 3.5, mucosal injury decreases rapidly corresponding to the decreasing pH-related pepsin activity. Together, the pH of the refluxate, frequency and duration of exposure define the extent of oesophageal injury. With an increased percentage of time during which the oesophagus is exposed to a pH <4, the severity of GERD increases subsequently. It is, therefore, of importance that, in reflux patients, the luminal and mucosal pH in gastric fundus, the mucosal pH in the gastric corpus and the luminal pH in the antrum is lower than in controls.[17]

In severe cases of GERD, bile reflux parallels acidic reflux which have a synergistic role.[18]

PATHOLOGICAL MECHANISMS CAUSING LARYNGOPHARYNGEAL REFLUX

Under physiological conditions, the upper aerodigestive tract is protected from gastric contents by the length of the oesophagus, its peristaltic and the upper oesophageal sphincter (UES). Experimental evidence in humans has shown that application of HCl close to the LES leads to an increase of the pharyngeal sphincter pressure, thereby protecting the otolaryngeal and the respiratory tract.[19] Reflux episodes into the oesophagus also cause an abrupt increase in upper oesophageal sphincter pressure. Interestingly, the duration of UES pressure increase was significantly longer in healthy subjects (25 s) than in GERD patients (15 s), indicating that UES tone duration is a physiological mechanism affected in GERD patients.

Willing et al.[20] have demonstrated that GER causes oesophageal distension which induces transient upper sphincter relaxations (TUESRs) in children. This study showed that 94% of TUESRs occurred within 4 s following oesophageal distension. These relaxations are most likely the mechanism underlying pharyngeal reflux, as the basal pressure of the upper oesophageal sphincter tone is not decreased in EERD children.[20]

Brief exposure to refluxate may not affect the oesophagus but can lead to mucosal irritation in the upper aerodigestive tract and lower airways. Serious effects on the mucosal surface are caused in the laryngeal region by reflux episodes at pH < 4. Thus, the otolaryngeal epithelium is more sensitive to acid-induced injury than the oesophageal epithelium.[3]

RISK FACTORS FOR GERD/EERD

Intrinsic factors

Slowed gastric emptying, impaired oesophageal clearance, increased postcibal gastric acidity, decreased salivation, and poor oesophageal tissue resistance to damage by acid and pepsin are intrinsic factors which dispose for GERD and possibly EERD. In addition, a genetic predisposition has been identified for EERD. Prematurity is also significantly associated with the amount of GER and may, therefore, cause GERD and EERD.[21]

External factors

An increased feeding volume leads to a combination of prolonged GER episodes and enhanced GER volume in both healthy infants and infants with reflux. In children, adolescents and adults, dietary habits like caffeine, fried food, fatty meats, and frequent consumption of tomato sauces increase the risk for GERD and EERD. Furthermore, exposure to second-hand tobacco smoke in young children as well as smoking in older children and adolescents can contribute to the development of EERD.[22]

AETIOLOGY OF OME

FUNCTIONS OF THE EUSTACHIAN TUBE

The eustachian tube has three primary functions: (i) pressure regulation of the middle ear; (ii) protection of the middle ear from nasopharyngeal secretions; and (iii) clearance of fluids that accumulate in the middle ear. Pressure regulation and the contributing effects on gas equilibration were regarded as the most important functions of the eustachian tube.[11]

PATHOGENESIS OF EFFUSION

Bluestone[11] stated that eustachian tube dysfunction is the most important factor in pathogenesis of OME and other middle ear diseases.

OM can result from impaired ventilation of the middle ear or entry of fluids coming from the nasopharynx into the middle ear by aspiration or insufflation or reflux. As the mucosa of the middle ear depends on a continuous supply of air via the eustachian tube from the nasopharynx, interruption of ventilation induces an inflammatory process that causes secretory metaplasia, impairs mucociliary transport, and leads to effusion of fluid into the tympanic cavity.[9] The metaplasia of the middle ear epithelium with proliferation of goblet cells and mucus glands, which causes hypersecretion of mucus, proceeds to accumulation of a mucin-rich viscous effusion in the middle ear cleft.[9]

ENDANGERED GROUPS OF PATIENTS

The high prevalence of OME in infants and young children may be attributable to the immaturity of the structure and function of the eustachian tube and the immaturity of the immune system.[11] Analysis of the effusion from OME revealed various bacteriological species including *Streptococcus pneumoniae*, *Haemophilus influenzea* and *Staphylococcus* spp.[23] Recently, the Gram-negative bacterium *Helicobacter pylori* has been discussed as a causative agent, but the relationship between *H. pylori* and OME is not completely understood.[24]

RISK FACTORS FOR OME DEVELOPMENT

A higher prevalence of middle ear infections and OME is attributable to overcrowding, poor hygiene, poor nutrition, passive smoking, high rates of nasopharyngeal colonization with potentially pathogenic bacteria and inadequate or unavailable health services.[9,11]

CONSEQUENCES OF OME

Formation of effusion can impair hearing and lead to hearing losses. Hearing impairment during the language-forming years causes difficulties with phonological awareness, word articulation, and development of receptive vocabulary. Even intermittent hearing loss may lead to inconsistent or partial auditory signals and, subsequently, interfere with normal speech and language development.

LINK BETWEEN OME AND REFLUX

PREVALENCE OF GERD/PHARYNGEAL REFLUX IN OTOLOGICAL DISORDERS

If OME is mainly or partially caused by EER, the prevalence of EER should be higher in patients with OME compared to healthy controls. Indeed, several studies revealed a significantly higher prevalence of GERD and pharyngeal acid reflux among patients who suffer from suspected reflux-associated otological disorders.[5,7,8,25] In patients with otolaryngeal symptoms suspected to have EERD, Koufman[3] observed an abnormal pH in the oesophagus in 62% and pharyngeal reflux in 30%. Using 24-h pH-metry. Velepic et al.[7] also documented pathological GER in 60% of patients with secretory, recurrent, or chronic OM.

In a small study of six children with suspected otalgia due to gastro-oesophageal reflux, all had pathological GER and were symptom-free following antireflux therapy.[8] Keles et al.[25] observed pharyngeal reflux in 48% of children with chronic otitis media but only in 8% of healthy controls.

Nevertheless, two large epidemiological studies showed that GER is not a causative agent in otitis media.[6,26] Unfortunately, El Serag et al.[26] studied only children older than 2 years, the children suffering from otolaryngeal disorders were older than the controls, and, importantly, not only cases with OME but all cases with OM were included. As OME is most common during the first 2 years of life and as the prevalence decreases with age, this might partially explain the lack of association. Despite this, the study by Carr et al.[6] included 99 infants younger than 2 years during ventilation tube insertion and found pathological reflux only in 7%.

SUCCESS OF ANTIREFLUX TREATMENT

In addition to a higher prevalence, improvement of otolaryngeal symptoms as a consequence of antireflux treatment would indicate a causative relationship. In a number of studies, otolaryngeal symptoms improved due to antireflux therapy in 60–100% of the cases and antireflux surgery in infants with otolaryngeal disorders led to partial or complete symptom relief.[3,8]

MECHANISM OF INTERACTION BETWEEN EER AND OME

A causative relationship between EER and OME requires that the gastric contents can reach the middle ear and, thereby, affect the mucosa. Observations obtained in animal and human studies indicate that this is possible.

GER occurs physiologically in neonates and infants during the first year of life and the frequency decreases with increasing age. In infants, GER is observed in 20%[27] with documented reflux into pharynx occurring in almost half of these children and nearly all reflux episodes in preterm babies. Due to the angle between nasopharynx and eustachian tube and the immaturity of the eustachian tube, gastric refluxate coming from the nasopharynx could possibly reach the middle ear. Inflammation of the nasopharynx and eustachian tube could follow and a disordered pressure equalization could result in eustachian tube dysfunction.[11] A prerequisite for this mechanism of interaction is that EER coming from the nasopharynx passes through the eustachian tube.

REFLUXATE COULD PASS THE EUSTACHIAN TUBE

Using a plasma pepsinogen ELISA, Tasker et al.[28] observed an increased amount of pepsins in the middle ear of infants with OME indicating reflux of gastric contents. This finding of increased pepsinogen levels in the middle ear was confirmed by others.[29] However, the specificity of the ELISA in middle-ear effusion is unclear, increased pepsin contents were not necessary related to increased GER symptoms[29] and the amount of pepsin in the middle ear of healthy humans remains unknown.

Recently, we have also demonstrated that GER reaches the middle ear in a Mongolian gerbil model using ear and larynx endoscopy and histology.[30]

A study on adult patients during the recovery phase from general anaesthesia provides no evidence that intranasally given radionuclide passes into the middle ear.[31] On the other hand, this study only investigated adults; therefore, in neonates and infants, where OME is commonest, the case may be different.

INJURY OF MIDDLE EAR EPITHELIUM

The eustachian tube is covered by ciliated respiratory epithelium. Multiple exposure of the tube to acidic pH values lower than 4 and pepsin might cause ciliostasis of this epithelium contributing to impaired mucociliary clearance. Direct experimental evidence has shown that transtympanic injection of a hydrochloric acid/pepsin solution or acid solution of the same concentrations as in the gastric juice led to increased eustachian tube opening pressure and impaired mucociliary clearance in rats.[32]

CONCLUSION

Taken together, it is possible that GER reaches the middle ear in infants and it has been demonstrated that gastric contents cause eustachian tube dysfunction, a main cause of OME. Several studies found a high prevalence of gastro-oesophageal or laryngopharyngeal reflux in infants with OME indicating a possible relationship. In addition, improvement of symptoms and findings of otolaryngeal disorders in patients treated with antireflux therapy suggest that extra-oesophageal reflux contributes to OME. Despite this, the causative relationship is not proven as yet. El Serag and Carr performed large studies which showed no increased prevalence of gastro-oesophageal reflux among infants with OM. Due to the high prevalence of both GER (occurring in 20% of infants) and OME (occurring 90% of all infants in the first 2 years of life), it is important to clarify if a possible causative relationship exists. On the other hand, the high prevalence of both disorders could hamper the examination of the association between them. Therefore, further evidence needs to be obtained in children.

CLINICAL FEATURES OF GERD AND EERD

REFLUX SYMPTOMS

Typical symptoms suggestive to GERD are common, including heartburn, epigastric pain, regurgitation, emesis, difficulties in swallowing, burping, rumination, chest pain and abdominal pain.[22] However, Koufman[3] found these typical GERD symptoms, including heartburn and regurgitation, in only 43% of the patients with otolaryngeal disorders caused by EER. Thus, these typical symptoms are often missing in patients with EERD, and variable symptoms may camouflage in other more common illnesses.

On the other hand, nearly one-third of otolaryngeal symptoms were suggested to result from GER. Thus hoarseness (71%), chronic cough (51%), dysphagia, frequent throat clearing (42%) or globus sensation (47%) are frequently attributable to EER.[2,3] In children and adolescents, breathing difficulties, hoarseness, dysphagia, emesis, throat clearing, early onset asthma, recurrent sinusitis and cough, headache, ear pain with and without recurrent otorrhoea or chronic otitis media have been observed as common symptoms of EERD. Infants affected by EERD symptoms often suffer from airway flow irritation, feeding or eating disturbances, otolaryngological symptoms or other constitutional symptoms.[22]

As extra-oesophageal symptoms caused by the refluxate may occur without the typical GERD symptoms (*e.g.* heartburn and regurgitation), high accuracy is required in the diagnosis of GERD as a possible cause of the symptoms.

DIFFERENCE PATTERN OF REFLUX DISEASE IN EERD AND GERD PATIENTS

The different symptoms presented by GERD and EERD patients may be attributable to the finding that patients with GERD mostly suffer from a supine nocturnal reflux combined with disorders of oesophageal motility, whereas EERD patients have upright day-time reflux and a normal oesophageal motility.[2] In reflux patients with chronic laryngeal symptoms, GER worsens in the upright position. Typical symptoms of GERD are uncommon among these patients. Moreover, it appears that patients with laryngeal reflux have a relatively good oesophageal acid clearance compared to GERD patients.[2] In addition, EERD patients have more laryngeal reflux but a similar degree of oesophageal reflux.[33]

DIAGNOSIS

OTITIS MEDIA WITH EFFUSION

OM should be classified as acute OM or OME. OME is defined as fluid in the middle ear without local or systemic illness. The two requirements for a diagnosis of acute otitis media are inflammation of, and fluid in, the middle ear.[11]

EXTRA-OESOPHAGEAL REFLUX DISEASE

For the diagnosis of EERD, a pathological degree of extra-oesophageal reflux correlated to otolaryngeal disorders is required. The causative relationship can be demonstrated by the association of symptoms to reflux episodes during pH-metry or impedance measurements. Another possibility is a successful therapeutic trial which eliminates or diminishes symptoms and/or findings. If otolaryngeal symptoms occur and EER is diagnosed, the association should be evaluated.

Laryngopharyngeal reflux can be diagnosed by evaluation of the patient's complete history, the head–neck examination, laryngoscopy, 24-h double or triple pH probe study, intraluminal impedance measurement, barium swallow, a therapeutic trial, and studies to diagnose other extra-oesophageal symptoms, such as pulmonary function.[2]

LARYNGEAL EXAMINATION

The laryngeal examination shows an inflamed pharynx with lymphoid hyperplasia (cobble-stoning), palatal and uvular oedema; characteristic dental erosion may occasionally be observed. Laryngeal findings are regarded as pathognomonic when lingual tonsillar hyperplasia, posterior glottic swelling (twice the normal anteroposterior width of the posterior glottis) and loss of the arytenoid architecture are visible. Two or more of these symptoms have a sensitivity of 87.5% and a specificity of 68% to predict reflux with 24-h pH probe, oesophagram, gastric scintiscan or oesophageal biopsy. Except for these laryngeal aspects, the physical examination is often normal.[22]

LARYNGOSCOPY

Laryngoscopic findings, that may be GERD-related, include erythema and oedema of the medial wall of the arytenoids, interarytenoid bar, and posterior pharyngeal cobble-stoning. A score has been developed on the basis of laryngoscopic findings that can help in documenting treatment efficacy.[3,34]

MONITORING pH

Dual probe 24-h pH monitoring

For the diagnosis of laryngopharyngeal reflux contributing to otolaryngeal disorders in both adults and children, dual probe 24-h pH monitoring is the gold standard, superior to endoscopy, single probe pH-metry, and barium studies.[12] Paediatric oesophageal pH monitoring is performed by transnasal placement of a standard micro-electrode into the lower oesophagus for continuous recording of the intra-oesophageal pH. The so-called reflux index, giving the percentage of time pH is less than 4, is a reliable and clinically useful measurement when obtained under standard conditions.

It is not necessary to perform oesophageal pH-metry if the diagnosis of GERD or EERD is already well established by symptoms or endoscopy. However, oesophageal pH-metry is very useful to document an association between symptoms and EER episodes.[1,35] The relationship between otolaryngeal symptoms and reflux can be detected if symptoms occur at the same time as episodes of EER.[35] Furthermore, oesophageal pH recordings in adults and paediatric patients are indicated if atypical symptoms of reflux occur, if suspected otolaryngeal manifestations (laryngitis, pharyngitis, chronic cough) of EERD are not improved by standard therapy with a twice-daily proton pump inhibitor (PPI)[36] and for the follow-up of patients treated surgically or medically.[35] In patients with otolaryngeal symptoms, it is important to use at least a dual probe technique for evaluating both upper oesophageal (or pharyngeal) and lower oesophageal acidification, as pH abnormalities may be limited to the upper oesophageal probe.[12] Due to a false-negative rate of 25%, the 24-h dual pH probe may be no better than the use of symptoms and the laryngeal examination.[22]

Bravo pH monitoring

A new alternative to standard pH probes is a wireless pH recording system (Bravo pH monitoring system; Medtronic, Shoreview, MN, USA). The small implantable capsule adheres to the oesophageal mucosa and transmits intraluminal data to a small receiver that the patient carries. After several days, the capsule spontaneously detaches; endoscopic retrieval is rarely necessary. The proposed advantage is a more representative profile as individuals are more likely to continue with normal activity during this type of pH recording. It has been used in adults and a small sample of children to get data of acid exposure in the oesophagus.[37] Until now, the size of the capsule has limited its use in paediatric patients, especially infants and young children.

However, all pH recording techniques are unable to detect the non-acidic reflux that occurs in the absence of pH changes. Due to a low degree of proton secretion, this non-acidic reflux is of particular importance in infants and young children. During the post-prandial period, hydrochloric acid is buffered by the neutralizing components of a meal, especially in milk-fed infants. Here pH monitoring can not detect reflux episodes in a group of patients frequently affected by OME.

In adult patients, duodenogastro-oesophageal reflux is known to be important for the pathogenesis of reflux oesophagitis, and occurs across the whole pH spectrum.[18] Moreover, severe forms of oesophagitis are related to an increased exposure of both gastric and duodenal reflux. The oesophageal mucosa is highly sensitive to this non-acidic reflux and, therefore, one may hypothesize that the respiratory epithelium of otolaryngeal structures is even more susceptible to this type of reflux. Consequently, it is of importance to document duodenogastro-oesophageal reflux in paediatric and adult patients.

METHODS TO DETECT NON-ACIDIC DUODENOGASTRO-OESOPHAGEAL REFLUX

Bilitec 2000

A useful method to measure bile contents in the oesophagus is bilirubin monitoring using the Bilitec sensor (Bilitec 2000; Synectics Medical, Stockholm, Sweden). Continuous monitoring of the absorbance of light allows the detection of bilirubin.[18]

Intraluminal impedance measurement

Another promising tool is intraluminal impedance measurement. This novel technique is based on the demonstration of fluid or gas in the oesophagus by changes in electrical conductance across pairs of electrodes placed into the oesophageal lumen. In combination with a pH electrode, this technique allows display of both acidic and non-acidic reflux. Intraluminal impedance measurement has the further advantage of giving additional information on direction of flow and bolus height. Oesophageal pH monitoring and impedance measurement in infants with reflux symptoms revealed that only 15% of all episodes were acidic; therefore, intraluminal impedance as a pH-independent technique seems appropriate for EER detection in infants.[38]

ENDOSCOPY

Among patients with typical GERD symptoms, endoscopy and biopsy can document the presence and severity of oesophagitis, strictures, Barrett's oesophagus and exclude other disorders. Direct visualization and biopsy may be indicated in children who present atypical symptoms or whose symptoms persist despite acid suppressive therapy.[3] Nevertheless, a normal appearance during endoscopy does not exclude histopathological changes. Therefore, oesophageal biopsy is recommended to detect microscopic oesophagitis and exclude a cause of oesophagitis other than GER.[1] Despite these advantages, oesophagoscopy is unreliable for the diagnosis of EERD, as oesophagitis may not be present even if severe otolaryngoscopy problems have already developed.

OTHER DIAGNOSTIC TOOLS

Other diagnostic tools include ultrasonography (which was found useful in the diagnosis of GERD), barium oesophagram (which occasionally shows reflux), and the gastric scintiscan (which reveals delayed gastric emptying highly associated with EERD on the 24-h pH probe).

Due to the safety of PPIs, a therapeutic approach of time-limited treatment for GER is useful to evaluate whether GER is causative for specific symptoms. For patients with suspected reflux-induced otolaryngeal disorders, a PPI therapy twice daily for 8–12 weeks is reasonable.[36]

THERAPY

OTITIS MEDIA WITH EFFUSION

In contrast to acute otitis media, OME should not be treated with an antibiotic. Effusion is likely to persist after the successful treatment of an acute OM, but a repeated treatment is not required as the fluid usually disappears within 3 months regardless of antibiotic treatment.

GERD/EERD

Acid-suppressive treatment
Life-style modifications may be effective to cure reflux disease but the majority of patients require pharmacological therapy. Healing of oesophageal injury and success of maintenance therapy depend on the time the gastric contents remain at pH 4.0 or more neutral. Using proton pump inhibitors, healing of lesions occurs more completely and in shorter time periods than observed using histamine-2 antagonists. The absence of serious adverse events of PPIs (combined with their high efficacy in healing and the low number of relapses) makes PPI treatment the first choice in maintenance of severe reflux disease in adults. PPIs have also clearly improved the therapeutic management for children with acid reflux with increasing evidence of their efficacy and safety.[1]

In studies with the PPIs omeprazole, lansoprazole, pantoprazole and esomeprazole, all were equally as effective and well-tolerated in therapy of

GERD. No significant differences between omeprazole, lansoprazole, pantoprazole and rabeprazole were found in improvement of symptoms and mucosal healing. The pharmacokinetics of these PPIs show higher metabolic capacity in children, with a maximum between 1–5 years;[39] elimination was reduced in babies under 6 months of age and, thereby, the antisecretory effect seems to be higher.[40] Therefore, in children older than 1 year, higher doses of proton pump inhibitors per kilogram are necessary since they metabolize these medications more quickly (compared to adults).

PPIs have to be administered prior to a meal to achieve full potency as the drug binds only to the proton pump of the activated parietal cell. The proton pump becomes maximally activated during the first meal after an overnight fast, so that PPI should be taken before breakfast. Unfortunately, it has been reported that nearly 70% of primary care physicians prescribed PPIs without any specific instructions or suggest it be taken before bedtime.[36]

If symptoms of GERD do not improve and for treatment of EERD, PPIs were found to be most effective when dosed twice daily, with the second dose taken before dinner. Laryngeal reflux often requires higher doses of antireflux treatment than typical cases of GERD;[2] as a result, the daily dose often has to be doubled compared to GERD patients. Therefore, it is appropriate to treat patients initially with high doses of antireflux medication to achieve healing, symptom relief and marked acid suppression. Later, the doses may be lowered until the lowest effective maintenance dose is reached. Caution is required as for GERD patients; it is known that decreasing the PPI dose after healing of symptoms and oesophagitis leads to rapid relapse of findings and symptoms. Beginning in early childhood, EERD may also require prolonged or even life-long treatment in certain cases.[2]

Promotility agents
Promotility agents (prokinetics) are lacking in predictable safety and efficacy. Metoclopramide, erythromycin, domperidone, baclofen and tegaserod maleate (Zelnorm; Novartis Pharmaceuticals USA, East Hanover, NJ, USA) have all been studied, but lack convincing data regarding value, although individual children may received benefit.[36]

Changes in dietary habits and life-style
Though the majority of patients require pharmacological therapy, patients should be educated regarding the factors that contribute to GER, as non-pharmacological measures could improve symptoms. Therefore, changes in dietary habits and life-style have to be considered. Many patients can identify foods that induce or worsen symptoms and they should be made aware of foods that frequently causes reflux – fatty meats, citrus fruits, tomato-based products, coffee (including decaffeinated), chocolate, and alcohol (particularly beer). Despite this, a recommendation to avoid all food that is potentially provocative is overly restrictive. To decrease the abdominal pressure, weight reduction in overweight patients, therapy of cough and other respiratory problems could be helpful. Smoke exposure, and food allergies are also associated with a higher frequency of GERD and EERD.[22,36] In infants, elimination of the soother and the feeding bottle after 9–12 months is helpful to diminish the risk of EERD. As many common medications like antihypertensives (calcium-channel blockers, nitrates),

bronchodilators (oral β_2-agonists), and psychotropic agents promote GER, it is important to evaluate the medication history.[36]

Key points for clinical practice

- Extra-oesophageal reflux (EER) is recognized as a causative agent in otorhinolaryngological disorders including pharyngitis, globus, subglottic stenosis, laryngitis and laryngeal carcinoma. Otitis media with effusion, rhinosinusitis, laryngomalacia and adenoidhypertrophy may also be attributable to EER.

- Otitis media with effusion is an asymptomatic middle-ear effusion persistent for at least 3 months.

- In most cases, reflux into the oesophagus occurs during transient relaxations of the lower oesophageal sphincter, induced by gastric distension.

- The tone of the upper oesophageal sphincter protects otolaryngeal structures from duodenogastric contents. Laryngopharyngeal reflux is probably caused by transient relaxations of this structure.

- Despite evidence of higher EER prevalence among children with otitis media with effusion (OME) in several studies and successful antireflux treatment for OME, two large studies found a lack of association between OME and reflux.

- Reflux coming from the nasopharynx can possibly pass into the eustachian tube. Hydrochloric acid, pepsin and eventually bile contents may cause dysfunction of the eustachian tube and contribute to formation of effusion.

- In contrast to typical reflux, symptoms like regurgitation and heartburn are only present in less than half of all EERD patients. These patients are often affected by hoarseness, frequent throat clearing, breathing disorders, asthma, chronic cough.

- Pathognomonic laryngeal findings for EER include lingual tonsillar hyperplasia, posterior glottic swelling (twice the normal anteroposterior width of the posterior glottis) and loss of the arytenoid architecture. Two of these symptoms have a high sensitivity for predicting laryngopharyngeal reflux.

- pH monitoring and impedance measurement can prove a causative relationship between EER and otolaryngeal disorders, if symptoms occur during investigation. A therapeutic trial leading to improving otolaryngeal symptoms and findings during antireflux treatment also indicates an association.

- Proton pump inhibitors are regarded as first choice in maintenance of reflux disease. To treat EERD patients effectively, it important that they receive higher doses and they should be requested to take proton pump inhibitors prior to a meal (breakfast, or breakfast and dinner).

References

1. Rudolph CD, Mazur LJ, Liptak GS *et al*. Guidelines for evaluation and treatment of gastroesophageal reflux in infants and children: recommendations of the North American Society for Pediatric Gastroenterology and Nutrition. *J Pediatr Gastroenterol Nutr* 2001; **32 (Suppl 2)**: S1–S31.
2. Koufman J, Sataloff RT, Toohill R. Laryngopharyngeal reflux: consensus conference report. *J Voice* 1996; **10**: 215–216.
3. Koufman JA. The otolaryngologic manifestations of gastroesophageal reflux disease (GERD): a clinical investigation of 225 patients using ambulatory 24-hour pH monitoring and an experimental investigation of the role of acid and pepsin in the development of laryngeal injury. *Laryngoscope* 1991; **101 (Suppl 53)**: 1–78.
4. Halstead LA. Role of gastroesophageal reflux in pediatric upper airway disorders. *Otolaryngol Head Neck Surg* 1999; **120**: 208–214.
5. Ulualp SO, Toohill RJ, Shaker R. Pharyngeal acid reflux in patients with single and multiple otolaryngologic disorders. *Otolaryngol Head Neck Surg* 1999; **121**: 725–730.
6. Carr MM, Poje CP, Ehrig D, Brodsky LS. Incidence of reflux in young children undergoing adenoidectomy. *Laryngoscope* 2001; **111**: 2170–2172.
7. Velepic M, Rozmanic V, Velepic M, Bonifacic M. Gastroesophageal reflux, allergy and chronic tubotympanal disorders in children. *Int J Pediatr Otorhinolaryngol* 2000; **55**: 187–190.
8. Gibson Jr WS, Cochran W. Otalgia in infants and children – a manifestation of gastroesophageal reflux. *Int J Pediatr Otorhinolaryngol* 1994; **28**: 213–218.
9. Paradise JL. Otitis media in infants and children. *Pediatrics* 1980; **65**: 917–943.
10. Teele DW, Klein JO, Rosner B. Epidemiology of otitis media during the first seven years of life in children in greater Boston: a prospective, cohort study. *J Infect Dis* 1989; **160**: 83–94.
11. Bluestone CD. Epidemiology and pathogenesis of chronic suppurative otitis media: implications for prevention and treatment. *Int J Pediatr Otorhinolaryngol* 1998; **42**: 207–223.
12. Jecker P, Orloff LA, Mann WJ. Extraesophageal reflux and upper aerodigestive tract diseases. *ORL J Otorhinolaryngol Relat Spec* 2005; **67**: 185–191.
13. Nelson SP, Chen EH, Syniar GM, Christoffel KK. Prevalence of symptoms of gastroesophageal reflux during childhood: a pediatric practice-based survey. Pediatric Practice Research Group. *Arch Pediatr Adolesc Med* 2000; **154**: 150–154.
14. Gold BD. Gastroesophageal reflux disease: could intervention in childhood reduce the risk of later complications? *Am J Med* 2004; **117 (Suppl 5A)**: 23S–29S.
15. Dent J, Dodds WJ, Friedman RH *et al*. Mechanism of gastroesophageal reflux in recumbent asymptomatic human subjects. *J Clin Invest* 1980; **65**: 256–267.
16. Masclee AA, de Best AC, de Graf R, Cluysenaer OJ, Jansen JB. Ambulatory 24-hour pH-metry in the diagnosis of gastroesophageal reflux disease. Determination of criteria and relation to endoscopy. *Scand J Gastroenterol* 1990; **25**: 225–230.
17. Quigley EM, Turnberg LA. Studies of luminal and mucosal pH in reflux esophagitis and antral gastritis. *Dig Dis* 1992; **10**: 134–143.
18. Orel R, Vidmar G. Do acid and bile reflux into the esophagus simultaneously? Temporal relationship between duodenogastro-esophageal reflux and esophageal pH. *Pediatr Int* 2007; **49**: 226–231.
19. Wallin L, Boesby S, Madsen T. The effect of HCl infusion in the lower part of the oesophagus on the pharyngo-oesophageal sphincter pressure in normal subjects. *Scand J Gastroenterol* 1978; **13**: 821–826.
20. Willing J, Davidson GP, Dent J, Cook I. Effect of gastro-oesophageal reflux on upper oesophageal sphincter motility in children. *Gut* 1993; **34**: 904–910.
21. Sutphen JL, Dillard VL. Effects of maturation and gastric acidity on gastroesophageal reflux in infants. *Am J Dis Child* 1986; **140**: 1062–1064.
22. Brodsky L, Carr MM. Extraesophageal reflux in children. *Curr Opin Otolaryngol Head Neck Surg* 2006; **14**: 387–392.
23. Brook I, Yocum P, Shah K, Feldman B, Epstein S. Microbiology of serous otitis media in children: correlation with age and length of effusion. *Ann Otol Rhinol Laryngol* 2001; **110**: 87–90.

24. Sudhoff H, Rajagopal S, Baguley DM *et al*. A critical evaluation of the evidence on a causal relationship between *Helicobacter pylori* and otitis media with effusion. *J Laryngol Otol* 2007; 1–7 [DOI 10.1017/S0022215107000989].

25. Keles B, Ozturk K, Gunel E, Arbag H, Ozer B. Pharyngeal reflux in children with chronic otitis media with effusion. *Acta Otolaryngol* 2004; **124**: 1178–1181.

26. El Serag HB, Gilger M, Kuebeler M, Rabeneck L. Extraesophageal associations of gastroesophageal reflux disease in children without neurologic defects. *Gastroenterology* 2001; **121**: 1294–1299.

27. Nelson SP, Chen EH, Syniar GM, Christoffel KK. Prevalence of symptoms of gastroesophageal reflux during infancy. A pediatric practice-based survey. Pediatric Practice Research Group. *Arch Pediatr Adolesc Med* 1997; **151**: 569–572.

28. Tasker A, Dettmar PW, Panetti M, Koufman JA, Birchall JP, Pearson JP. Reflux of gastric juice and glue ear in children. *Lancet* 2002; **359**: 493.

29. Lieu JE, Muthappan PG, Uppaluri R. Association of reflux with otitis media in children. *Otolaryngol Head Neck Surg* 2005; **133**: 357–361.

30. Sudhoff H, Bucker R, Groll C, Shagdarsuren S, Dazert S, Schreiber S. Tracing of gastric reflux into the middle ear in a Mongolian gerbil model. *Otol Neurotol* 2007; **28**: 124–128.

31. Ayanoglu E, Uneri C, Turoglu T, Dogan V. Reflux of nasopharyngeal content into middle ear through the eustachian tube. *Eur Arch Otorhinolaryngol* 2004; **261**: 439–444.

32. Heavner SB, Hardy SM, White DR, McQueen CT, Prazma J, Pillsbury III HC. Function of the eustachian tube after weekly exposure to pepsin/hydrochloric acid. *Otolaryngol Head Neck Surg* 2001; **125**: 123–129.

33. Jacob P, Kahrilas PJ, Herzon G. Proximal esophageal pH-metry in patients with 'reflux laryngitis'. *Gastroenterology* 1991; **100**: 305–310.

34. Belafsky PC, Postma GN, Koufman JA. The validity and reliability of the reflux finding score (RFS). *Laryngoscope* 2001; **111**: 1313–1317.

35. Colletti RB, Christie DL, Orenstein SR. Statement of the North American Society for Pediatric Gastroenterology and Nutrition (NASPGN). Indications for pediatric esophageal pH monitoring. *J Pediatr Gastroenterol Nutr* 1995; **21**: 253–262.

36. Lowe RC. Medical management of gastroesophageal reflux disease. *GI Motility online* 2006 [DOI 10.1038:gimo54].

37. Ahlawat SK, Novak DJ, Williams DC, Maher KA, Barton F, Benjamin SB. Day-to-day variability in acid reflux patterns using the BRAVO pH monitoring system. *J Clin Gastroenterol* 2006; **40**: 20–24.

38. Wenzl TG, Moroder C, Trachterna M *et al*. Esophageal pH monitoring and impedance measurement: a comparison of two diagnostic tests for gastroesophageal reflux. *J Pediatr Gastroenterol Nutr* 2002; **34**: 519–523.

39. Zhao J, Li J, Hamer-Maansson JE *et al*. Pharmacokinetic properties of esomeprazole in children aged 1 to 11 years with symptoms of gastroesophageal reflux disease: a randomized, open-label study. *Clin Ther* 2006; **28**: 1868–1876.

40. Hoyo-Vadillo C, Venturelli CR, Gonzalez H *et al*. Metabolism of omeprazole after two oral doses in children 1 to 9 months old. *Proc West Pharmacol Soc* 2005; **48**: 108–109.

James Keir Helen Beer Terry Jones

7

Proteomics and genomics of head and neck squamous cell carcinoma

Head and neck squamous cell carcinoma (HNSCC) is the sixth commonest cancer in the world. In the UK, the incidence of HNSCC per annum is 12–13/100,000.[1,2] Despite recent developments in treatment, prognosis has not improved in the last 15 years. The 5-year survival rate still remains around 50%.[3]

HNSCC develops as a consequence of the dysregulation of many different molecular pathways. The aberrations of the molecular pathways involved occur due to the sequential acquisition of DNA mutations, which ultimately result in a growth advantage over normal surrounding cells. Such mutations manifest as either down-regulation of tumour suppressor genes and/or up-regulation of oncogenes or other genes which promote cellular transformation or tumour metastasis. In addition to the role of DNA mutation, there is increasing evidence that infective agents, for example human papilloma virus (HPV), and epigenetic mechanisms may also play a central role in malignant transformation of epithelial cells of the upper aerodigestive tract.[4] In numerous case series, HPV genomic DNA has been consistently detected in 20% of HNSCCs and about 50% of oropharyngeal or tonsillar SCCs.[5–10] These HPV-positive patients less frequently have a p53 mutation and more frequently have a basaloid morphology and better survival.[5,11]

With the exception of nasopharyngeal carcinoma, the mainstay of treatment of HNSCC involves radiotherapy, surgery with or without postoperative

James Keir MRCS DOHNS (for correspondence)
Specialist Registrar in Otolaryngology, Royal Liverpool Children's Hospital, Alder Hey, Liverpool, UK
E-mail: jameskeir@hotmail.com

Helen Beer MRCS(Ed)
Specialist Registrar in Otolaryngology, Countess of Chester Hospital, Chester, UK

Terry Jones BSc(Hons) MD FRCS
Senior Lecturer and Honorary Consultant in Head and Neck Cancer Surgery/Otolaryngology, School of Cancer Studies, University of Liverpool, Liverpool, UK
E-mail: terry.jones@liverpool.ac.uk

radiotherapy or cisplatin-based chemoradiotherapy, or chemoradiotherapy alone. HNSCC is typically considered as a homogeneous tumour group, despite the fact that tumours arise from several major anatomical sub-sites within the upper aerodigestive tract. Whilst tumours may be histopathologically identical, they are often genetically disparate and exhibit variable biological behaviour and response to treatment between and within anatomical sub-sites.[12]

Until recently, research into the molecular basis of HNSCC (and other solid tumours) has concentrated on individual genes or gene pathways and their products, in an attempt to elucidate underlying mechanisms of transformation or to identify clinically relevant biomarkers. Moreover, whilst significant advances have been made in our understanding of discrete molecular pathways involved in tumour formation, the complexity of the integrated mechanisms involved in tumorigenesis has ensured that the investigation of individual genes or their products as biomarkers of biological behaviour or treatment response has been disappointing. Consequently, treatment decisions for patients presenting with HNSCC are still based on clinical, radiological and pathological parameters. Currently, outside on-going research protocols, no molecular markers are routinely used in treatment decision making.

Only since the development of newer, more powerful, analytical techniques (which allow investigation of the genome, transcriptome or proteome as a whole) has it been possible to investigate the multiple and concurrent mechanisms which may be involved. These techniques hold considerable promise for the development of strategies which may allow early diagnosis (especially of recurrent disease), predict biological behaviour and treatment response whilst identifying novel therapeutic targets. It is also hoped that they will provide information that will finally allow us to understand the molecular mechanisms involved in the development of HNSCC. These newer techniques are included in the disciplines of genomics and proteomics.

PROTEOMICS

Proteins are the ultimate product of gene expression. The proteome comprises all the proteins present in a cell (or biofluid) at a given point in time. It has been estimated that a typical mammalian cell will contain 10,000–20,000 different proteins resulting in ~10^9 individual protein molecules. The copy number of individual protein species varies widely from less than 20,000 molecules of a given protein per cell (rarest) to 100×10^6 copies (most abundant). Any protein which has in excess of 50,000 copies is generally considered to be abundant. In a typical mammalian cell, about 2000 proteins will fall into this category. The proteome contains proteins of huge diversity which are able to co-ordinate and facilitate all of the functions required for cellular homeostasis. Particular functions of cellular proteins include biochemical catalysis, the maintenance of cellular structure, cell movement, cellular transport, cell signalling, immunity and storage.[13]

Following malignant transformation, the protein profile of a cancer cell will differ from its wild-type progenitor. As proteins are the effectors of cellular behaviour, proteins expressed following malignant transformation are likely to orchestrate unregulated tumour growth, direct tumour invasion and subsequent metastatic seeding, dictate the interaction of tumour cells with surrounding stromal tissues and cells and, ultimately, dictate biological behaviour and treatment response.

Proteomic studies are important because of the link the proteome provides between the genome and the biochemical capability of the cell. It can be argued that study of the proteome is more representative of cell function than study of the transcriptome (and by inference the genome). Whilst the transcriptome will indicate which genes are active, it is not a good indicator of protein function as mRNA content does not necessarily correlate well with protein expression. Neither does it take into account the rate of protein degradation nor the regulation of protein function by post-translational modification.

The term proteomics is a generic term, describing a diverse collection of techniques designed to study protein activity, concentration, modification, activation and localisation as well as the interaction of proteins within complexes. However, it is increasingly being used to describe techniques used to study the composition of a proteome. This technique should, strictly speaking, be called protein profiling or expression proteomics.

EXPRESSION PROTEOMICS

Expression proteomics most commonly relies on the combined use of two techniques – two-dimensional gel electrophoresis (2-D GE) and mass spectrometry (although antibody or lysate arrays may be used in place of 2-D GE). Each technique has, for many years, been used routinely in research laboratories, however, expression proteomics has only become possible since their combination with mass spectrometry following technological advancements.

Two-dimensional gel electrophoresis

Individual proteins within a mixture can be separated by making use of the chemical and physical differences of the constituent proteins. Two-dimensional gel electrophoresis (2-D GE) employs a combination of two common protein separation strategies. The first, which separates proteins on the basis of mass, uses sodium dodecyl sulphate (SDS), a detergent, which, when mixed with protein, denatures the tertiary structure of the protein and confers a negative charge which is proportional to the polypeptide length. When this mixture is applied to one end of an agarose gel and an electric current is applied across it, the proteins will migrate on the basis of size towards the positive electrode; the smallest migrating fastest and, therefore, farthest. The second technique involves isoelectric focusing. This strategy relies on the fact that individual protein species have different net electrical charge. Thus when a protein mixture is run, by applying an electric current across an agarose gel which contains chemicals that create a pH gradient, individual protein species will migrate along the gel until they reach their isoelectric point, i.e. at a point when the net charge is zero. In 2-D GE, proteins are first separated by isoelectric focusing. Following this, the gel is soaked in SDS and rotated through 90° prior to repeating the separation, this time according to size. Following this, staining of the gel reveals a complex pattern of spots, each representing a single protein species. These are scanned by densitometers and the image analysed by software packages for spot detection

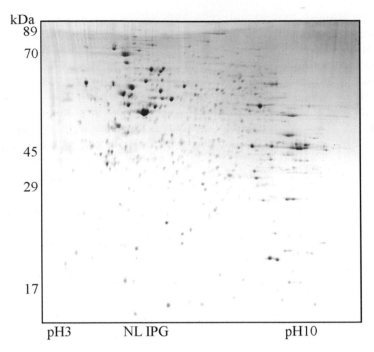

Fig. 1 Two-dimensional gel electrophoresis protein spot profile of squamous cell line.

and quantification;[14] several thousand protein species may be separated in a single gel (Fig. 1).

The novel application of this technique follows comparison of gels derived from different protein mixtures. Differences in patterns and intensity of spots can be identified. These differences relate to the differential expression of a particular protein species between the proteomes being studied.

The second stage of this process uses mass spectrometry to enable identification of the protein species represented by the spot(s) of interest.

Mass spectrometry

The steps involved in mass spectrometry (MS) are conceptually simple. The protein species defined by an individual spot following 2-D GE can be extracted from the polyacrylamide-gel following excision of the spot of interest. The extracted protein is then digested into smaller polypeptide fragments using a sequence-specific protease, *e.g.* trypsin. This results in a mixture of varying length polypeptides (typically 5–75 amino acids in length) derived from the originally purified protein. The next stage is to ionize these polypeptides, using a source of ionizing radiation. Following this, the charged polypeptides are propelled along a mass analyser by an electric or magnetic field during which they are separated on the basis of their mass/charge (m/z) ratio. Differing m/z ratios manifest as differences in 'time-of-flight' (TOF) as the ionized polypeptides pass from the ionizer to the detector. This ensures that individual polypeptide species are separated temporally and spatially prior to impact on a detector. The data are visualised as a spectrum from which the m/z profile of the polypeptide mix may be compared with the vast databases created a consequence of the Human Genome Project. The databases contain the sequences of all putative human proteins, ultimately allowing identification of the parent protein.

The combination of these techniques allows the comprehensive screening of comparative proteomes, enabling the identification and characterisation of specific proteins which are either up- or down-regulated during malignant transformation or during contrasting phenotypic expression. These data can be correlated with genomic data derived from the same tissue to identify specific, perhaps novel, pathways which contribute to the clinical outcomes identified.

COMPARISON OF PROTEOMES

Over recent years, in addition to the more precise protein identification strategies outlined above, technological advances in the speed, accuracy and sensitivity of mass spectrometry have meant that it can now be used to assess complex protein samples derived from tissue or biofluids. Furthermore, the completion of the Human Genome Project has allowed the development of databases containing the protein sequences of all supposed human proteins. Therefore, significant effort and resources are now being directed towards attempts to define clinically meaningful protein profiles of disease states, which can be used as reliable biomarkers of clinical outcome. The ultimate goal of these strategies is the development of proteomic 'fingerprints' whose presence or absence correlates tightly with disease state or tumour behaviour.

The requirement to analyse the vast quantities of complex data generated by these techniques has necessitated the development of advanced bioinformatic algorithms. Such techniques use statistical modelling to distinguish sources of experimental error due, for example, to signal to noise effects and, the random sampling of low abundance proteins, from the detection of true biological variation.

As biomarkers do not currently exist, these strategies are increasingly being investigated as to their applicability in HNSCC.

The most commonly used MS techniques used to compare proteomes include matrix-assisted laser desorption and ionization (MALDI) and surface enhanced laser desorption and ionization (SELDI).

MALDI

MALDI is normally used to analyse relatively simple peptide mixtures and utilises laser energy to ionize mixtures of proteins and/or polypeptides. Laser energy applied directly to protein mixtures fragments the protein and, therefore, a dry, crystalline matrix (often a UV-radiation absorbing organic acid) is mixed with or applied to the sample. The matrix absorbs the brunt of laser energy thereby minimising protein fragmentation, before transferring lower energy levels to the proteins or peptides which ionizes them. However, the induced ionization is not uniform and is dependent on both the chemical characteristics of the individual polypeptides or proteins and their relative abundance. Smaller proteins and polypeptide chains are more easily ionized and, consequently, most proteins detected by MALDI have an m/z of less than 50 kDa. MALDI typically incorporates a time-of-flight (TOF) mass analyser in which intact proteins or peptides are separated on the time it takes them to

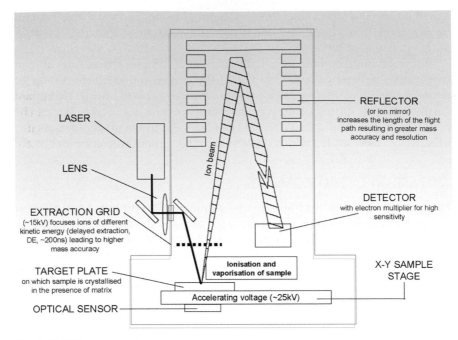

LASER

LENS

REFLECTOR
(or ion mirror)
increases the length of the flight
path resulting in greater mass
accuracy and resolution

Ion beam

DETECTOR
with electron multiplier for high
sensitivity

EXTRACTION GRID
(~15kV) focuses ions of different
kinetic energy (delayed extraction,
DE, ~200ns) leading to higher
mass accuracy

TARGET PLATE
on which sample is crystallised
in the presence of matrix

OPTICAL SENSOR

Ionisation and
vaporisation of sample

Accelerating voltage (~25kV)

X-Y SAMPLE
STAGE

Fig. 2 MALDI mass spectrometry.

traverse a flight tube and strike the detector with the numbers of ions striking the detector being counted (Fig. 2).[15,16] An important limitation of MALDI is that it is a semiquantitative technique that has limited sensitivity for low abundance proteins. The m/z signal detected not only depends on the amount of polypeptide present but also its ionization characteristics. Therefore, rather than detecting specific protein species, MALDI allows the comparison of relative abundance of a given protein species within two different lysates. Despite these drawbacks, the technique allows the assessment of intact proteins within whole tissue with minimal sample preparation and volume. It is able to cope with a high throughput and is able to separate 10^2–10^3 polypeptides from a complex mixture making it useful to study biological samples comparatively.

SELDI
SELDI utilises a chemically modified surface on a ProteinChip which has affinity for polypeptides with certain biophysical properties, *e.g.* hydrophobic affinity, net electric charge or the ability to bind a given metal. This enables the partial purification of complex protein mixtures, such as a serum or tumour lysate. Following adsorption, the surface is washed to remove any proteins that bind poorly. Following this, the bound proteins are liberated and analysed as described for MALDI. Whilst this ensures partial purification of the initial sample, SELDI binding is not specific, and reproducibility is an acknowledged technical problem. Moreover, this lack of specificity may result in proteins of interest being eluted out at the initial purification stage, especially if their binding characteristics dictate that they are in competition for surface binding domains with more abundant protein species.

Early diagnosis/screening

Published observational studies indicate that patients whose diagnosis of cancer is delayed may require more extensive treatment and experience poorer outcomes.[17] In particular, the diagnosis of small tumours before the development of regional metastases is associated with dramatically improved survival and decreased treatment related morbidity. Both clinical and radiological assessments are dependent on the presence of 1–2 cm of tumour growth (representing approximately 10^9 cells) and, therefore, are only moderately sensitive and specific in detecting early head and neck cancer.[12] The use of proteomics to identify markers in serum or saliva could aid early detection of small lesions and may even provide a screening strategy for high-risk groups. Speight et al.[18] have suggested that screening of high-risk groups (such as male smokers and drinkers over the age of 40 years) may be cost effective. Furthermore, expression profiling could be used to monitor the progression of pre-malignant lesions (especially in those areas that are difficult to assess without a general anaesthetic), as well as contributing to the assessment of response to treatment and the detection of recurrent HNSCC during follow-up. This may be particularly important as recurrent or metachronous tumours are not uncommon.[19]

Several research teams have attempted to identify biomarker profiles in the serum in patients with HNSCC. Sidransky et al.[20] obtained MALDI spectra on sera from 143 controls and 99 patients with high stage (grade III–IV) HNSCC. The data from two-thirds of the patients and controls were used to generate a training set. Following this, the data from the remaining one-third of patients and controls (the test set) was then assessed in light of the training set outcomes. Over 280,000 features were identified in the resulting spectra. This number was subsequently reduced to a more manageable 2800 features by considering only one in every 100 data points. Many of the distinguishing peaks were in a range of 0–21 kDa. Following comparison of training and test sets, 45 features were identified which enabled patients with HNSCC to be distinguished from controls with a sensitivity of 73% and specificity of 90%.

Wadsworth et al.[21] used spectra from sera of 99 patients with HNSCC and 127 controls which included 25 'healthy' smokers. No comment was made on the stage of HNSCC in this group. Again, a test set and training set were utilised to produce a best profile features of which were shared by 90.7% of patients with HNSCC in the training set and which correctly identified 83.3% of patients with HNSCC in the test set. Similarly, Soltys et al.[22] analysed proteomic spectra from the serum of 113 patients with HNSCC and 104 controls. A training set of 56 patients with HNSCC and 53 controls correctly identified HNSCC with a sensitivity of 63% and a specificity of 77%, whilst a sensitivity of 68% with a specificity of 73% was established for the detection of patients within the test set which comprised 57 HNSCC patients and 52 controls. A weakness of this study, acknowledged by the authors, is that most of the HNSCC patients had stage III–IV tumours at diagnosis and, therefore, had involved neck nodes at diagnosis. Given that the aim was to detect patients with HNSCC at an earlier stage, it is recognised that studies comprising patient groups with early stage disease will need to be conducted in order to attempt to answer this question.

Gourin *et al.*[23] studied serum samples in 78 patients with HNSCC and in 68 healthy controls. The spectral peaks they identified as being differentially expressed between the two groups allowed detection of patients with HNSCC with a sensitivity of 82%, a specificity of 76%, and a positive predictive value of 83% (slightly lower values than those seen by Wadsworth *et al.*[21]). Furthermore, the spectral differences identified, could distinguish between tumour from different primary sites in 83% of oral cavity, 81% of oropharyngeal and 88% of laryngeal tumours. Several limitations to the study were noted; these include small sample size in the validation set, and statistically significant epidemiological differences between the HNSCC and control groups.

Cheng *et al.*[24] obtained serum MALDI spectra for 57 patients with oral cancer and compared them with 29 healthy controls. Eighteen patients had early stage disease (stage I or II) whilst 39 had advanced disease (stage III–IV). Six spectral markers were identified that differentiated between cancer patients and controls, but no spectral differentiation was demonstrable between patients with different disease stage. One marker in particular, a 2664-Da polypeptide (identified as a fragment of the fibrinogen α-chain) had the highest sensitivity (100%) and specificity (97%) in detecting patients. While this study identifies a potentially valuable biomarker, it needs to be established whether this marker is present in the serum of patients with benign or premalignant conditions such as leukoplakia, or other types of cancer.

It is obvious that these data will need further validation in larger studies, particularly as the numbers of patients in each study were relatively small when compared with the number of data points available. Selection of fewer data points, a necessary requirement to create more manageable datasets, inevitably increases the risk of selecting spurious *m*/*z* peaks by chance. As well as this, because of the plethora of potential host- and tumour-related confounding factors, control groups for HNSCC studies are difficult to construct. It is possible that the effects of such confounding factors on proteomic spectra might be profound although this has yet to be established.[25]

PROGNOSIS AND TREATMENT RESPONSE

Despite heterogeneity in tumour behaviour, no sub-classification of HNSCC currently exists.[26] Proteomic profiles obtained using MALDI on non-small cell lung cancer tissue from tumours of a similar stage and histological grade allow their classification based on the presence or absence of nodal metastases with 75% accuracy; it was also possible to identify patients with worse survival outcomes.[27] Should such discrimination prove possible in HNSCC, the benefits are obvious, as individual patient treatment strategies may be tailored accordingly. For example, depending on the sub-site of the primary tumour, up to 30% of patients with clinical and radiological node negative HNSCC may have occult metastases.[28–30] Therefore, currently, up to 70% of patients with node-negative disease receive unnecessary therapy to ensure a minority who are truly at risk are adequately treated.[25] Were it possible to identify those at true risk reliably, the unnecessary treatment received by the majority of this patient group could be avoided.

Similarly, it is well established that HNSCC exhibits wide variation in response to radio- and/or chemotherapy.[31] It may, therefore, be possible to identify tumour protein profiles which are indicative of susceptibility or resistance to given treatment regimens or combinations thereof. It may also prove possible from such studies to identify novel therapeutic targets. Several preliminary studies[32–35] have attempted to do just this, by specifically seeking up- or down-regulated proteins in HNSCC which may in future be used as novel therapeutic and/or diagnostic markers.

However, any putative biomarker(s) would need to be validated in large, multicentre, randomised, controlled trials. Thus, despite the huge promise offered by this technology, there is a long way to go before it is incorporated into day-to-day clinical practice.

GENOMICS

Previous research has concentrated on techniques used to identify single, or at most several, gene mutations that may contribute to tumour phenotype. Given that there are probably multiple genetic mutations involved in the tumorigenesis of HNSCC, methods that provide a more global assessment of tumour genotype could have potentially wide-ranging, valuable clinical applications. The development of DNA microarray and Gene Chip technology now offers the possibility of analysing global gene expression patterns which may allow the detection of premalignant lesions likely to develop into invasive carcinoma, confirm the presence or absence of disease, predict clinical outcome and treatment response, thereby enabling the targeting of optimal management.

Practical constraints of this technology include its high cost and the quantity of the data. Genomic experiments typically result in the detection of thousands of variables which are often measured against tens of cases. False-positive results and data overfitting are, therefore, significant problems.[36]

DNA MICROARRAY TECHNOLOGIES

Microarrays generally involve samples of DNA with known sequences being spotted and immobilised onto a substrate, most commonly on a glass microscope slide or silica slide only 1–2 cm square. RNA isolated from samples of interest is reverse transcribed into cDNA and labelled with spectrally distinct fluorescent dyes (Fig. 3). In small or necrotic tumours, only very small amounts (5–100 ng)[26] of RNA might be retrievable, necessitating amplification. Because the dyes used to label RNA have distinct characteristics, two labelled cDNA samples may be pooled and hybridised in a single microarray which has been spotted with cDNA from thousands of genes, each representing one gene. Strands of cDNA in the pooled samples hybridise to their complementary sequence immobilised on the substrate, and any unbound cDNA is washed off. The ratio between fluorescent signal intensities of the two dyes at a particular position is representative of the relative abundance of the corresponding mRNA and, therefore, gene expression in the samples. In other techniques, target RNA is labelled with a single fluorophore and hybridised onto the immobilised DNA probes. The degree of fluorescence at each

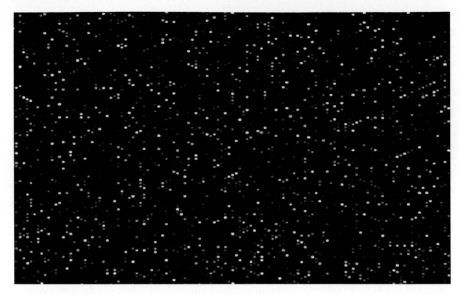

Fig. 3 A DNA microarray in analysis of gene expression.

immobilised DNA probe determines gene expression. It has been found that long-term storage of samples even without evidence of RNA degradation affected prediction accuracy. This suggests that time intervals for processing of samples from procurement to gene expression analysis should be regulated.[26]

Statistical tools are used to identify the vast quantities of data generated by a single microarray experiment. These analyses may be supervised or unsupervised. Supervised analysis selects genes that are associated with 'supervising' parameters or conditions such as absence or presence of metastasis. The analysis, therefore, uses the supervising parameter to create an expression profile that gives the highest prediction accuracy for genes that distinguish the two groups.[26,37] After a predictive gene list has been generated from a training set, the results are confirmed by a leave-one-out cross validation and, ultimately, by analysis of an independent cohort of patient samples.[38]

Unsupervised techniques analyse the data only on the gene expression pattern regardless of specific characteristics of the tissue being examined. It is possible to segregate different histological tumour types or tumours from the normal tissue in which they arose based on these analyses and even allow identification of tumour subtypes.

CLINICAL APPLICATIONS OF MICROARRAY TECHNOLOGY

Prediction of progression in HNSCC

Further understanding of the sequence of genetic alterations from normal epithelia to malignant transformation may allow the detection of lesions destined to progress, enabling their therapeutic targeting to prevent progression. Ha *et al.*[39] have described expression arrays used to examine malignant, premalignant and histopathologically normal mucosa obtained from the upper aerodigestive tract of patients or normal controls. A total of 334 genes were associated with progression from normal to premalignant; however, only 23 genes were found to be associated with progression from premalignant to malignant. In other words, the majority of genetic alterations are found to occur prior to conversion to invasive malignancy.

Prediction of metastasis

Chung et al.[40] analysed gene expression to predict metastases in 60 primary and previously untreated HNSCCs. Several supervising parameters were used to increase the accuracy. Pathological staging of nodal metastasis was found to give the greatest accuracy as a supervising parameter, especially when analysed on the basis of anatomical subsites. When examining oropharyngeal, hypopharyngeal and laryngeal SCCs, a predictive accuracy of 83% was achieved. Cromer at al.[41] examined hypopharyngeal SCCs to compare three groups of patients: (i) those who developed metastases; (ii) those who did not develop metastases; and (iii) those who had a local recurrence within 3 years of treatment. Using 168 gene targets, metastatic prediction accuracy was 92%, suggesting, as might be expected, that sub-site analyses improves accuracy. Roepman et al.[37] investigated the predictive strength of 102 differentially expressed genes (i.e. those which had been up-regulated or down-regulated) for lymph node metastases from 82 primary SCCs of the oral cavity and oropharynx. An overall predictive accuracy of 86% was achieved compared with a clinical staging accuracy of 68%. The predictor genes in this study were compared with the data set of another group.[40] They found that 45 of the 102 genes were present on their microarray; however, none overlapped with their predictive gene list.

In contrast, a further study[42] analysed gene expression in normal mucosa and in the tumour tissue of patients presenting with HNSCC with and without distant metastases (> 3 tumour-positive lymph nodes). Despite identifying 150 differentially expressed genes in HNSCC with versus without metastasis, none of the differential expression patterns achieved statistical significance between the tissues examined and therefore, an expression profile could not be identified.[42]

The non-concordance of predictive gene expression patterns is common in microarray studies, especially if different platforms and data mining tools are used. Whilst it is commonly presumed that these differences are likely to represent differences in experimental design or data analysis, it may be that these are true differences which relate to the underlying biology. The practical issues of microarray experiments have been investigated by members of the Toxico-genomics Research Consortium who identified the sources of error and data variability among seven different laboratories and across 12 microarray platforms. They determined that these variations could be minimised by use of a common platform and standard procedures.[43] Further research on larger sample sizes needs to be carried out to standardise methods, which should then be validated by large clinical trials in other independent centres.

MOLECULAR CLASSIFICATION OF HNSCC

Belbin et al.[44] performed a preliminary study attempting to sub-type tumour tissue extracted from 17 patients with HNSCC. The microarray profile from these tumour samples was compared with the expression profile of normal human epithelial keratinocytes (HNEKs). The HNEKs were obtained commercially and were not from the head and neck mucosa although the authors reported they were close in nature to the tumour cell type. The study identified 906 genes that enabled subclassification of the tumour tissue into two distinct groups. On the basis of the genomic data, 16 patients were equally divided into two distinct groups. However, the expression profile resulting from one tumour resisted its inclusion into either group. These two groups differed in tumour differentiation and cause specific survival ($P = 0.057$). A further study by Chung et al.[39] enabled HNSCCs to be divided into four clinically distinct groups on the basis of the genomic expression patterns. The study was unsupervised and included 60 HNSCC samples. The classification was independent of the primary tumour site, histological differentiation and stage but had statistically significant differences in recurrence-free survival and overall survival. Ginos et al.[45] analysed 41 HNSCC tumours and compared them with normal oral mucosa samples in an attempt to identify biomarkers of locoregional recurrence. A gene set was identified that was associated with invasion, metastasis and recurrence. It is suggested that recurrence, at least in part, is due to gene mutations of the primary tumour; therefore, if this recurrence signature is detectable, management may be tailored accordingly.

TARGETED MANAGEMENT

As with proteomics, it is hoped that genomic profiles of HNSCCs susceptible to different treatment modalities may be identified. For example, in non-small cell lung cancers, the EGFR inhibitor gefitinib was found to be relatively ineffective for therapy when the entire population of patients was evaluated. However a subgroup of patients with EGFR mutations had a remarkable response.[46,47] It has been suggested that gene expression analyses may be used to identify gene mutations responsible for angiogenesis, apoptosis, deregulated signalling or proliferative pathways. It is further proposed that this may then be used to direct specific targeted therapies with regards to chemotherapeutic agents. The ability to study multiple gene mutations may also direct attempts to correct or treat key genetic aberrations on a pan-genomic scale using, for example, targeted gene therapy. Hanna et al.[48] described a microarray expression profile of 1187 tumour-related genes in radiation-resistant and radiation-sensitive tissue biopsies. A radiation-sensitive tumour was defined as no evidence of tumour, whereas radiation-resistant tumour was defined as < 40% decrease in tumour size at the end of 6 weeks of treatment with a total of 68–70 Gy. Sixty of the 1187 tumour-related genes were identified as being predictors of response to radiation. This observation was subsequently confirmed by the successful prediction of radiation response in two tumours.

CONCLUSIONS

Proteomics and genomics hold great challenges and possibilities for the future. The quantity of data analysed using these techniques is unprecedented and the technology will need to develop standardised acquisition and analysis of data, which are subsequently validated by independent centres. The potential bias in these studies is large and includes technical factors such as time required to conduct an assay, the batch of reagents used, the skill levels of the technician and the bio-informatics tools used to assess the data. Confounding factors such as age, gender, cancer stage, tumour histology and treatment delivered in a small sample size is a particular problem in HNSCC. Many of the present studies do not correct for this and a minimum head and neck data set should be established to allow appropriate interpretation. A further example of controversial methodology that is applicable to both genomics and proteomics is whether all of the tissue harvested is analysed. It is a potentially confounding factor if infiltrating stromal, vascular and inflammatory cells are included in analysis and, therefore, it is argued that laser capture microdissection should be used to ensure that only tumour cells are analysed. Others disagree and argue that the non-epithelial components of tumours may contribute significantly to the overall clinical behaviour and should, therefore, be included. Once standardisation has occurred, any clinical application will then require large multicentre, randomised, controlled trials. If these challenges can be overcome, then revolutionary change in the management of HNSCC may prove possible.

Key points for clinical practice

- Previous research of the molecular basis of head and neck squamous cell carcinoma (HNSCC) has concentrated on individual markers; however, proteomics and genomics are potentially powerful tools that could be used to study changes in the proteome or genome as a whole.

- The use of proteomics to identify markers in serum or saliva could aid screening and early detection of HNSCC. It could also be used to monitor progression of premalignant lesions and response to treatments.

- While several potential proteomic biomarkers have been identified, none have reached a stage at which they may be clinically applicable.

- Despite heterogeneity in tumour behaviour, no sub-classification of HNSCC currently exists. Proteomics and genomics may be potentially useful in differentiating any sub-classification.

- Gene expression analysis has been used with some success to predict metastasis particularly when analysed on the basis of anatomical subsites. Further studies are required for validation and investigation of non-concordance of results between studies.

- Genomic profiling could be used in targeting treatment modalities and small-scale studies have taken place.

- Proteomics and genomics have great potential to revolutionise the treatment of HNSCC; however, many challenges remain before it may be used in the clinical setting.

References

1. Parkin DM, Laara F, Muir CS. Estimates of the worldwide frequency of 16 major cancers in 1980. *Int J Cancer* 1988; **41**: 19–36.
2. Vokes EE, Weichselbaum RR, Lippmann, Hong WK. Head and neck cancer. *N Engl J Med* 1993; **328**: 184–194.
3. Forastiere A, Koch W, Trotti A, Sidransky D. Head and neck cancer. *N Engl J Med* 2001; **345**: 1890–1900.
4. Fan CY. Genetic alterations in head and neck cancer: interactions among environmental carcinogens, cell cycle control and host DNA repair. *Curr Oncol Report* 2001; **3**: 66–71.
5. Gillison ML, Koch WM, Capone RB *et al*. Evidence for a causal association between human papillomavirus and a subset of head and neck cancers. *J Natl Cancer Inst* 2000; **92**: 709–720.
6. Fouret P, Martin F, Flahault A *et al*. Human papillomavirus infection in the malignant and premalignant head and neck epithelium. *Diagn Mol Pathol* 1995; **4**: 122–127.
7. Paz IB, Cook N, Odom-Maryon T *et al*. Human papillomavirus (HPV) in head and neck cancer. An association of HPV 16 with squamous cell carcinoma of Waldeyer's tonsillar ring. *Cancer* 1997; **79**: 595–604.
8. Ringstrom E, Peters E, Hasegawa M *et al*. Human papillomavirus type 16 and squamous cell carcinoma of the head and neck. *Clin Cancer Res* 2002; **8**: 3187–3192.
9. Klussmann JP, Weissenborn SJ, Wieland U *et al*. Human papillomavirus-positive tonsillar carcinomas: a different tumor entity? *Med Microbiol Immunol (Berl)* 2003; **192**: 129–132.
10. Strome SE, Savva A, Brissett AE *et al*. Squamous cell carcinoma of the tonsils: a molecular analysis of HPV associations. *Clin Cancer Res* 2002; **8**: 1093–1100.
11. Schwartz SR, Yueh B, McDougall JK, Daling JR, Schwartz SM. Human papillomavirus infection and survival in oral squamous cell cancer: a population based study. *Otolaryngol Head Neck Surg* 2001; **125**: 1–9.
12. Rodrigo JP, Ferlito A, Suarez C *et al*. New molecular diagnostic methods in head and neck cancer. *Head Neck* 2005; **27**: 995–1003.
13. Brown TA. *Genomes 3*. New York: Garland Science, 2007.
14. Srinivas P, Srivastava S, Hanash S, Wright GL. Proteomics in the early detection of cancer. *Clin Chem* 2001; **47**: 1901–1911.
15. Aebersold R, Mann M. Mass spectrometry-based proteomics. *Nature* 2003; **422**: 198–207.
16. Pandey A, Mann M. Proteomics to study genes and genomes. *Nature* 2000; **405**: 837–846.
17. Kowalski LP, Franco EL, Torloni H *et al*. Lateness of diagnosis of oral and oropharyngeal carcinoma: factors related to the tumour, the patient and the health professionals. *Eur J Cancer B Oral Oncol* 1994; **3**: 167–173.
18. Speight PM, Palmer S, Moles DR *et al*. The cost-effectiveness of screening for oral cancer in primary care. *Health Technol Assess* 2006; **10**: 1–144, iii–iv.
19. Spitz MR. Epidemiology and risk factors for head and neck cancer. *Semin Oncol* 1994; **21**: 281–288.
20. Sidransky D, Irizarry R, Califano JA *et al*. Serum protein MALDI profiling to distinguish upper aerodigestive tract cancer patients from control subjects. *J Natl Cancer Inst* 2003; **95**: 1711–1717.
21. Wadsworth JT, Somers KD, Stack Jr BC *et al*. Identification of patients with head and neck cancer using serum protein profiles. *Arch Otolaryngol Head Neck Surg* 2004; **130**: 98–104.
22. Soltys SG, Le QT, Shi G *et al*. The use of plasma surface-enhanced laser desorption/ionization time of flight mass spectrometry proteomic patterns for detection of head and neck squamous cell cancers. *Clin Cancer Res* 2004; **10**: 4806–4812.
23. Gourin CG, Zhong-Sheng X, Yan Han *et al*. Serum protein profile analysis in patients with head and neck squamous cell carcinoma. *Arch Otolaryngol Head Neck Surg* 2006; **132**: 390–397.
24. Cheng A, Chen L, Chien K *et al*. Oral cancer plasma tumour marker identified with bead-based affinity fractionated proteomic technology. *Clin Chem* 2005; **51**: 2236–2244.
25. Yarbrough WG, Siebos RJC, Liebler D. Proteomics: clinical applications for head and neck squamous cell carcinoma. *Head Neck* 2006; **28**: 549–558.
26. Chung CH, Levy S, Yarbrough WG. Clinical applications of genomics in head and neck cancer. *Head Neck* 2006; **28**: 360–368.

27. Yangiasawa K, Shyr Y, Xu BJ et al. Proteomic patterns of tumour subsets in non-small cell lung cancer. Lancet 2003; 362: 433–439.
28. Ambrosch P, Bricbeck U. Detection of nodal micrometastases in head and neck cancer by serial sectioning and immunostaining. Oncology 1996; 10: 1221–1226.
29. Becker MT, Shores CG, Yu KK, Yarbrough WG. Molecular assay to detect metastatic head and neck squamous cell carcinoma. Arch Otolaryngol Head Neck Surg 2004; 130: 21–27.
30. Coatesworth AP, MacLennnan K. Squamous cell carcinoma of the upper aerodigestive tract: the prevalence of microscopic extracapsular spread and soft tissue deposits in the clinically N0 neck. Head Neck 2002; 24: 258–261.
31. Miura K, Suzuki S, Tanita J et al. Correlated expression of glutathione S-transferase-pi and c-Jun or other oncogene products in human squamous cell carcinomas of the head and neck: relevance to relapse after radiation therapy. Jpn J Cancer Res 1997; 88: 143–151.
32. Sewell DA, Yuan CX, Robertson E. Proteomic signatures in laryngeal squamous cell carcinoma. ORL J Otorhinolaryngol Relat Spec 2007; 69: 77–84.
33. Koike H, Uzawa K, Nakashima D et al. Identification of differentially expressed proteins in oral squamous cell carcinoma using global proteomic approach. Int J Oncol 2005; 27: 59–67.
34. Kato H, Uzawa K, Onda T et al. Down-regulation of 1D-myo-inositol 1,4,5-triphosphate 3-kinase A protein expression in oral squamous cell carcinoma. Int J Oncol 2006; 28: 873–881.
35. Melle C, Ernst G, Schimmel B et al. Biomarker discovery and identification in laser microdissected head and neck squamous cell carcinoma with ProteinChip technology, two-dimensional gel electrophoresis, tandem mass spectrometry and immunohistochemistry. Mol Cell Proteomics 2003; 2: 443–452.
36. Tinker AV, Boussioutas A, Bowtell DDL. The challenges of gene expression microarrays for the study of human cancer. Cancer Cell 2006; 9: 333–339.
37. Roepman P, Wessels LF, Kettelarij N et al. An expression profile for diagnosis of lymph node metastasis from primary head and neck squamous cell carcinomas. Nat Genet 2005; 37: 182–186.
38. Wu TD. Analysing gene expression data from DNA microarrays to identify candidate genes. J Pathol 2001; 195: 53–65.
39. Ha PK, Benoit NE, Yochem R et al. A transcriptional progression model for head and neck cancer. Clin Cancer Res 2003; 9: 3058–3064.
40. Chung CH, Parker JS, Karaca G et al. Molecular classification of head and neck squamous cell carcinomas using patterns of gene expression Cancer Cell 2004; 5: 489–500.
41. Cromer A, Carles A, Millon R et al. Identification of genes associated with tumorigensis and metastatic potential of hypopharyngeal cancer by microarray analysis. Oncogene 2004; 23: 2484–2498.
42. Braakhuis BJM, Senft A, Bree R et al. Expression profiling and prediction of distant metastases in head and neck squamous cell carcinoma. J Clin Pathol 2006; 59: 1254–1260.
43. Bammler T, Beyer RP, Bhattacharya S et al. Standardizing global gene expression analysis between laboratories and across platforms. Nat Methods 2005; 2: 351–356.
44. Belbin TJ, Singh B, Barber I et al. Molecular classification of head and neck squamous cell carcinoma using cDNA microarrays. Cancer Res 2002; 62: 1184–1190.
45. Ginos MA, Page GP, Michalowicz BS et al. Identification of a gene expression signature associated with recurrent disease in squamous cell carcinoma of the head and neck. Cancer Res 2004; 64: 55–63.
46. Paez JG, Janne PA, Lee JC et al. EGFR mutations in lung cancer: correlation with clinical response to gefitinib therapy. Science 2004; 304: 1497–1500.
47. Lynch TJ, Bell DW, Sordella R et al. Activating mutations in the epidermal growth factor receptor underlying responsiveness of non-small-cell lung cancer to gefitinib. N Engl J Med 2004; 350: 2129–2139.
48. Hanna E, Shrieve DC, Ratanatharathorn V et al. A novel alternative approach for prediction of radiation response of squamous cell carcinoma of the head and neck. Cancer Res 2001; 61: 2376–2380.

David F. Hall William B. Coman

8

Vaccines and immunotherapy in head and neck cancer

Along with improvements in sanitation, vaccination revolutionised public health and is one of the most effective interventions against disease. The modern techniques of vaccination began with the inoculation or variolation which was practised in China from the 10th century and involved the deliberate infection of patients with powdered smallpox scabs (either by snorting or scratching the skin).[1] The technique reached Europe via Constantinople and was widely practised in the West until the early 1800s when Jenner's technique of inoculation with the much safer cowpox virus became popular.

The term 'vaccination' was first used by Edward Jenner in 1796 and is derived from the original Latin term for the cowpox virus *variolae vaccinae* (vaccinus from vacca; a cow) which he used in his smallpox inoculations. Jenner's observation that milkmaids were protected from smallpox if they had previously been infected with the cowpox virus led him to inoculate his patients successfully with this benign non-fatal strain.

Jenner is credited as the father of the 'smallpox vaccine' due to his efforts in spreading the use of vaccination and his work was the foundation for future vaccination programmes that would eventually see the eradication of smallpox in 1977.

Traditionally, there are considered to be four main vaccine types but a number of other innovative vaccines have recently reached the market or are in development (Table 1). In general, vaccines are considered to be prophylactic with the aim of either preventing or decreasing the effect of infection by

David F. Hall BSc(Hons) (NSW) MBBS(Qld) (for correspondence)
ENT Registrar, Department of Otolaryngology, Head and Neck Cancer Unit, The Princess Alexandra Hospital, Woolloongabba 4102, Queensland, Australia
E-mail: dfh74@hotmail.com

William B. Coman AM MD
Professor in Otolaryngology, Department of Otolaryngology, Head and Neck Surgery, The Princess Alexandra Hospital and University of Queensland, Woolloongabba 4102, Queensland, Australia
E-mail: drcoman@powerup.com.au

Table 1 Vaccine types

Killed	killed micro-organisms, *e.g.* influenza, cholera, hepatitis A, bubonic plague
Live attenuated	disabled micro-organisms, *e.g.* yellow fever, MMR
Toxoids	inactivated, toxic compounds from micro-organisms, *e.g.* tetanus, diphtheria
Subunit	fragments of micro-organisms, *e.g.* hepatitis B, human papilloma virus
Conjugated	combine parts of micro-organism to more immunogenic substance such as protein/toxins. *e.g.* HIB
Recombinant vector	combines physiology of one organism with DNA of another
DNA vaccination	insertion and expression of pathogen DNA into human or animal cells

pathogens. The term is now more broadly used and includes cancer or tumour vaccines, a type of immunotherapy designed as therapeutic interventions.

IMMUNOTHERAPY

Immunotherapy refers to a range of treatments that are effected by modulating the immune system and can include inducing, enhancing or suppressing the immune response. Cancer immunotherapy attempts to activate the immune system and enhance the body's innate defence against malignant tumours, thereby preventing the development of cancer or mediating the regression of established disease. In general, cancer immunotherapy can be classified as active or passive and specific or non-specific (Table 2).

This rapidly expanding group of therapies incorporates the use of cytokines (such as interferons, interleukins and colony stimulating factor) and monoclonal antibodies, and also includes tumour vaccines, the focus of this review.

OVERVIEW OF A TUMOUR VACCINE

A number of different approaches have been employed in the search for effective cancer vaccines including, but not limited to, autologous T-cell

Table 2 Immunotherapy definitions

Active immunotherapy	the induction of the immune response through application of immunogenic tumour antigens such as peptides, proteins, tumour cells or tumour lysates
Passive immunotherapy	indicates a transfer of immune effector molecules or immune cells
Specific	the ability to induce (active) or transfer (passive) tumour antigen-specific molecules or cells
Non-specific	the stimulation of the immune system using substances that activate or enhance immune cell function regardless of antigen specificity

transfer, modified and unmodified autologous tumour cells, tumour cell lysates, tumour peptides and antigens, heat-shock proteins, DNA, dendritic cells and virus-like particles. Therapies employing these techniques are in various stages of development; however, although early experiments and exhaustive animal studies have demonstrated the promising potential of vaccine-based approaches in the treatment of cancer, to date success in clinical trials involving a range of human malignancies has been limited. At present, three approaches warrant further review and are of particular relevance in head and neck cancer: (i) vaccines using viral-like particles; (ii) T-cell based adoptive transfer; and (iii) dendritic cell based immunotherapy.

This chapter will review currently used and developing immunotherapies based on each of these approaches and will outline their relevance in head and neck squamous cell carcinoma (HNSCC).

HEAD AND NECK SQUAMOUS CELL CARCINOMA

Head and neck cancer is a common malignancy affecting over 500,000 people world-wide.[2] The term refers to the group of primary tumours that arise from the mucosa of the upper aerodigestive tract (oral cavity, pharynx and larynx) and also includes lymphatic metastases to regional lymph nodes in the neck. The vast majority of these cancers are squamous cell carcinomas; however, in practise, the term is synonymous with head and neck squamous cell carcinoma (HNSCC).

Tobacco and alcohol are the most common risk factors for head and neck cancer accounting for the vast majority of tumours.[3] Other risk factors include betel-nut chewing, chronic trauma and the human papilloma virus.

Head and neck squamous cell carcinoma often presents management challenges to the treating team. Despite advances in the treatment of HNSCC over the last 40 years, overall survival has not changed significantly and for all-comers 5-year survival remains approximately 50%.[4] Considering the morbidity associated with the disease process, its treatment and the poor but variable prognosis, there is an urgent need for the development of new therapeutic techniques. Immunotherapies may form part of this evolving treatment armamentarium and will likely be used in conjunction with established therapies such as surgery, chemotherapy and radiotherapy.

HUMAN PAPILLOMA VIRUS

Papilloma viruses are a diverse group of double-stranded DNA viruses that infect epithelial cells in mammals, birds and reptiles.[5] They are composed of a non-enveloped icosahedral capsid (outer protein shell) containing a genome of approximately 8000 base pairs. The viral genome encodes two structural proteins (L1 and L2) and a number of non-structural proteins (E1, E2, E4, E5, E6, E7) necessary for gene expression, replication and for packaging into virus particles.[6]

Over 100 different papilloma viruses infect humans and these human papilloma viruses (HPVs) have been classified based on nucleotide sequence homology and order of discovery. From the HPV subtypes identified, approximately 40 have been consistently found to infect mucosal epithelium. Of these, only a small number appear of clinical significance. These HPV infections are commonly classified by their location – anogenital, non-genital cutaneous and non-genital mucosal.

It is also common to categorise HPV types into level of risk based on their carcinogenic potential. High-risk types (including 16, 18, 45, 31, 33, 52 and 58) are associated with cervical and anogenital cancers while low-risk types (including 6 and 11) are responsible for benign warts and papilloma. Work continues on the role of probable high-risk and undetermined-risk subtypes.[7]

Natural immune response to HPV is weak, generating only low antibody titre levels. The neutralising antibodies produced are generally of IgG type and are usually directed against the L1 virus capsid protein.[8] Despite these low and sometimes undetectable levels of antibodies, the vast majority of HPV infections are cleared from the body with few, if any, clinical symptoms. There is some evidence to suggest that previous infection with certain subtypes of HPV offers future protection from that subtype.[8]

To initiate infection, HPV particles must first penetrate the epidermis, usually through a defect in the stratified epithelium, so as to gain access to the basal cells where the virus is then maintained. The virus life-cycle proceeds from here and can result in HPV carcinogenesis, mediated by the replication proteins E6 and E7. These two oncoproteins interact with p53 and pRB inducing proliferation and malignant transformation.

ROLE OF HPV IN HNSCC

HPV is well established as a necessary factor in nearly all cancers of the cervix as well as most vaginal and anal cancer. There is now mounting evidence that HPV also contributes to a subset of head and neck squamous cell carcinomas. The link was first suggested in 1983 by Syrjanen *et al*.[9] and has recently been corroborated by further epidemiological and molecular evidence.[10]

Although a recent meta-analysis showed that HPV DNA was found in up to 26% of all HNSCCs, there is strong evidence that HPV has an affinity for the mucosa of the oropharynx (and in particular the tonsil) where HPV DNA is detected in over one-third of lesions.[11,12] The most prevalent type of HPV found in these HNSCC tumours is HPV 16 (up to 95%) and HPV 18, while other HPV types are rarely detected.[11]

Clinically, HPV-positive HNSCC patients are younger (by approximately 5 years) and are more likely to be non-drinkers and non-smokers than HPV-negative HNSCC patients. There is also emerging evidence that HPV-positive HNSCC has a markedly improved prognosis compared with tobacco- and alcohol-related HNSCC.[10]

HPV infection is mainly considered a sexually transmitted disease and, as with cervical cancer, certain sexual behaviours have been associated with a higher risk of developing HPV-positive HNSCC. Factors include number of sexual partners, history of genital warts and performance of oral sex.

HPV VACCINES IN HNSCC

Therapies aimed at treating existing HPV infections are in development; currently, the role of the HPV vaccine in HNSCC is in preventing initial infection and, thereby, hopefully reducing the incidence of HNSCC.

At present, there are two HPV vaccines on the market – Gardasil (from Merck) and Cervarix (from GlaxoSmithKline). Both are based on virus-like particle (VLP) technology. Although there were multiple contributors in both the US and Australia, both vaccines are based on break-through work performed by Frazer and Zhou at the University of Queensland.[13] In 1991, they produced non-infectious virus-like particles using the papilloma virus capsid protein L1. Subsequent work demonstrated that these L1-based VLPs were capable of producing neutralising antibodies.[14–17]

The two vaccines differ in the number of HPV types they cover and in their method of production. The Merck vaccine, Gardasil, is a quadrivalent vaccine (covering HPV subtypes 6, 11, 16 and 18) produced from recombinant yeast (*Saccharomyces cerevisiae*). GlaxoSmithKline's Cervarix is a bivalent vaccine containing VLPs to mimic HPV 16 and HPV 18 and is produced using recombinant baculovirus in insect cells. Both vaccines include an aluminium adjuvant (to boost immunogenicity) that, in combination with the VLPs, produces an antibody response more potent than from HPV infection.

Clinical trials using both of these vaccines have demonstrated an antibody response in nearly 100% of those vaccinated with no serious vaccine-related side-effects. An octavalent vaccine (which expands the coverage to include HPV types 31, 45, 52 and 58 as well as 6, 11, 16 and 18) is currently in clinical trials.

It is now likely that a subset of oropharyngeal HNSCC is related to HPV infection. What remains to be shown is what role, if any, the new HPV vaccines have in the prevention and treatment of these lesions as no specific clinical trials have yet addressed this question. Even though the benefit is some time away, head and neck surgeons should involve themselves in the current discussions about the HPV vaccine as it is likely that wide-spread vaccination will eventually lead to a decline in the incidence of HNSCC. Issues which must be addressed include which vaccine to use, who and when to vaccinate and how often.

DENDRITIC CELL BASED THERAPIES

Originally described by Paul Langerhans in 1868 as 'branched skin cells resembling neurons', dendritic cells are derived from haemopoietic bone marrow progenitor cells. These antigen-presenting immune cells are found throughout the skin (where they are called Langerhans cells) and aerodigestive tract. Dendritic cells (DCs) reside as immature precursors in the peripheral tissues where they are often exposed to foreign antigens. These immature DCs pick up and process antigens and then migrate to lymph nodes. As part of this process, the dendritic cell matures and up-regulates expression of major histocompatibility complexes and adhesion molecules. They also become potent secretors of T-cell chemokines. On arrival in lymph nodes, DCs deliver the antigens to naïve T cells via major histocompatibility complexes, thereby initiating a cascade of T-cell activation.

DCs are a heterogeneous population of cells grouped into two main types – myeloid DCs and plasmacytoid DCs. This differentiation is based on phenotype (level of expression of CD11c and CD123) and function.[18]

Due to their crucial role in adaptive immunity, DCs have long been considered a possible basis for the development of an effective tumour vaccine. However, tumours are generally weakly immunogenic and so such therapy involves the use of *ex vivo* primed autologous DCs to induce an effective antitumour immune response.

Evolving research is addressing the challenges faced in the development of DC vaccines including the ideal source of DCs (peripheral blood DCs or *ex vivo* maturation of DC precursors), the best culture conditions (fetal calf serum-free media versus autologous serum) and the most appropriate antigen loading techniques – peptides, tumour parts (cells, cell lysates or DC-cell fusions), viral vectors, DNA or mRNA.

DC-based vaccines against a range of human malignancies including malignant melanoma, multiple myeloma, non-Hodgkin's lymphoma, renal tract malignancies and gastrointestinal malignancies have been trialed. Results have been mixed but they have shown that DC-based tumour vaccines are safe, generally well tolerated, and have minimal side-effects.

DENDRITIC CELL THERAPIES IN HNSCC

In HNSCC, research has shown improved prognosis in those tumours with a higher DC infiltrate. Such observations have been followed by promising results using DCs in human head and neck cell lines but, as yet, no clinical trials of DCs in HNSCC have been performed.

Wang et al.[19] have investigated the effect of a dendritic cell vaccine against a tongue SCC cell line (Tca8113) and demonstrated that tumour cell lysate pulsed DCs were able to induce a T-cell reaction against Tca8113 *in vitro* and inhibit tumour growth in nude mice. Recently, Jeong et al.[20] were able to protect mice from developing SCC tumours by vaccinating them with DCs educated with apoptotic SCC tumour cell lines. This suggests a possible role for DC therapy as not only a therapeutic vaccine but also as a prophylactic intervention for individuals at increased risk of HNSCC.[20]

EPSTEIN–BARR VIRUS

Epstein–Barr virus (EBV) was first identified in 1964 by Epstein, Achong and Barr during their work on Burkitt's lymphoma.[21] Further research soon identified this member of the herpes virus family as the cause of infectious mononucleosis[22] and EBV has since been implicated in a range of other diseases including post-transplant lymphoproliferative disorders, lymphoma and nasopharyngeal carcinoma.

EBV belongs to the gamma herpes virus family and is an enveloped virus containing a double-stranded DNA genome wrapped around a toroid-shaped protein core. This DNA core is surrounded by an icosahedral capsid and tegument. The virus encodes a set of lytic cycle genes (expressed during primary infection and during secretion of infectious virus) and a small group of latent proteins including EBV nuclear proteins (EBNAs) 1, 2, 3A, 3B, 3C and the latent membrane proteins (LMPs) 1, 2A and 2B23.

There are two different strains of EBV (Types 1 and 2) distinguished by variations in the genes that encode nuclear antigens. The two types also differ in their distribution with Type 1 predominating in Western countries and a mix of both Types 1 and 2 being found in Africa and Papua New Guinea. Humans are the sole natural host for both types of EBV and the virus infects more than

90% of the world's adult population, usually initially in early childhood or adolescence. After primary infection, which is often asymptomatic[24] but can in some cause glandular fever, individuals remain life-long carriers and, in most cases, the virus remains in equilibrium with its host.

Transmission of EBV is via saliva and primary infection occurs in the epithelium of the oropharynx.[25] This initial acute infection, which requires the activation of EBV lytic cycle proteins, proceeds to latent infection of B-lymphocytes in the oropharyngeal lymphoid tissue and then to persistence of the virus in circulating memory B-cells.

In a small number of carriers, latent infection can lead to the development of malignancies and these cancers have been classified based on their degree of expression of EBV latent proteins as either latency I (one protein expressed), II (several) or III (all expressed).

NASOPHARYNGEAL CARCINOMA

Nasopharyngeal carcinoma (NPC) is an uncommon carcinoma of the nasopharyngeal epithelium usually arising from the lateral nasopharyngeal recess (fossa of Rosenmüller) with an annual incidence that can range from < 1 per 100,000 in most parts of the world up to 50 per 100,000 in some parts of Southeast Asia.[26] Other areas with a significant incidence of NPC include Alaska, Greenland, North Africa and some Mediterranean countries. Men are affected more than women (approximately three to one) and the disease exhibits a bimodal peak onset (30–40 and 50–60).

The aetiology of NPC is multifactorial and includes: genetic predisposition (A2, B17 and Bw46, Cantonese Chinese), environmental (nitrosamines in salted fish, alcohol and tobacco) and viral (EBV).

EBV AND NASOPHARYNGEAL CARCINOMA

The World Health Organization classifies NPC into Types 1–3 (keratinising, non keratinising and undifferentiated carcinoma) and EBV is most closely associated with Types 2 and 3 in which up to 90% of patients have IgA antibodies to early antigen and viral capsid antigen. Studies have demonstrated clonal expansion of unique EBV DNA in NPC suggesting that a single EBV infected cell may be the initiating factor in the development of NPC.[27] Other characteristic histological features of NPC include the presence of a rich lymphocyte infiltrate.

As with all EBV-related malignancies, latent infection is crucial to carcinogenesis; in NPC, a type II latency pattern is seen in which there is an intermediate level of viral gene expression with limited expression of EBNA-1, LMP-1, LMP-2, EBER-transcripts and BamH1 A RNAs.[23]

NASOPHARYNGEAL CARCINOMA IMMUNOTHERAPY

Despite several problems which have hampered development of an effective immunotherapy for NPC (lack of expression of immunodominant EBV proteins and the immunosuppressive environment established by the malignancy), there are a number of features that make NPC an attractive target for immunotherapy:

1. Unlike the majority of human malignancies, in NPC the viral non-self targets LMP and EBNA1 are present; although these proteins are not immunodominant, they can be recognised by the immune system.

2. Also, unlike many human tumours, NPC exhibits MHC class I and TAP expression which facilitates presentation of antigen to cytotoxic T-cells.[28,29]

3. It has been shown that NPC cell lines are susceptible to lysis by EBV-specific cytotoxic T-lymphocytes (CTLs).

4. It is certain that cytotoxic T-lymphocytes are the major effector mechanism in controlling EBV infection (CTL-based adoptive transfer is known to cure post-transplant lymphoproliferative disease.

5. NPC immunotherapy is based on a large body of highly developed immunological literature.

6. It is likely that successful immunotherapy for NPC will be applicable to Hodgkin's lymphoma.

ADOPTIVE IMMUNOTHERAPIES FOR NASOPHARYNGEAL CARCINOMA

Adoptive therapy can be autologous or allogenic and involves the *ex vivo* activation of EBV-specific cytotoxic T lymphocytes (CTLs) with EBV epitopes. This therapy was initially developed over 10 years ago for the treatment of post-transplant lymphoproliferative disease (PTLD) and has since been utilised for a range of EBV-associated malignancies. Recently, the first clinical trials using EBV-specific cytotoxic T lymphocytes to treat advanced NPC patients were published.[30,31] These two small phase 1 studies each dosed 10 patients using between 2 and 23 autologous CTL infusions per patient. Although several patients did not respond, a combination of short- and long-term remissions (between 11–27 months) and partial responses among the majority of participants suggests the need for larger clinical trials possibly including stage I and II NPC patients with less extensive disease in whom complete long-term remission may be more likely.

Several such clinical trials are currently underway. In Brisbane, Australia at the Queensland Institute of Medical Research and the Princess Alexandra Hospital, Moss and Coman are performing a Phase I clinical trial of adoptive transfer of CTLs specific for EBV latent membrane proteins 1 and 2. A second trial to be run in Hong Kong and Brisbane will use a polytope of multiple CTL LMP1 and LMP2 epitopes encoded within a replication-deficient strain of adenovirus 5. Other groups have put LMP2 in to a viral vector and this trial is also underway.

Although promising results from preliminary clinical trials demonstrate the potential for EBV-specific CTL adoptive immunotherapy to assist in the treatment of NPC, it is unlikely to have wide-spread applications. Adoptive therapies must be individually made and require significant laboratory expertise and resources. As such, they are not feasible for use in many NPC-endemic areas. They are usefully in helping improve our understanding of NPC and EBV immunology and may also offer insights into the development of an effective EBV vaccine. Such a vaccine would aim to prevent the development of NPC and other EBV-related diseases, would be more cost effective and more widely available.

CONCLUSIONS

Immunotherapies are a relatively new, but rapidly expanding, group of treatments that may benefit head and neck cancer patients. Currently, their main applications in otolaryngology are in head and neck SCC and NPC; however, as our knowledge of the immune system and its role in malignancy increases, immunotherapy may be included as a treatment option for other rarer head and neck cancers.

Key points for clinical practice

- Vaccine: an antigenic preparation used to establish immunity to a disease.

- Immunotherapies can be active or passive and specific or non-specific and aim to modulate the immune system to prevent or treat disease.

- Human papilloma virus (HPV)-related head and neck squamous cell carcinoma (HNSCC) is most common in the oropharynx and is most often caused by high-risk HPV 16 and HPV 18.

- Dendritic cells can be used to prime the immune system by activating T cells and may eventually be used in a range of human malignancies.

- Nasopharyngeal carcinoma is an attractive target for immunotherapy and some initial promising results using adoptive therapy suggest that a more universally applicable vaccine could be developed.

ACKNOWLEDGEMENTS

The authors thank Dr David Chin, Dr Glen Boyle and Professor Denis Moss for their comments and suggestions during the preparation of this manuscript.

References

1. Temple R. *The Genius of China: 3000 Years of Science, Discoveries and Invention.* New York: Simon and Schuster, 1986.
2. Stewart BW, Kleihues P. *World Cancer Report.* Geneva: International Agency for Research on Cancer, 2003; 232–236.
3. Blot WJ, McLaughlin JK, Devesa SS, Fraumeni Jr JF. Cancers of the oral cavity and pharynx. In: Schottenfeld D, Fraumeni Jr JF. (eds) *Cancer Epidemiology and Prevention.* New York: Oxford University Press, 1996; 666–680.
4. Forsatiere A, Koch W, Trotti A, Sidransky D. Head-and-neck cancer. *N Engl J Med* 2001; **345**: 1890–1900.
5. Doorbar J. The papillomavirus life cycle. *J Clin Virol* 2005; **32 (Suppl)**: S7–S15.
6. Howely PM, Lowy DR. Pappilomaviridae. In: Knipe DM, Howley PM. (eds) *Field's Virology,* 5th edn. Philadelphia, PA: Lippincott Williams and Wilkins, 2007; 2299–2354.
7. Munoz N, Boach FX, de Sanjose S *et al.* Epidemiologic classification of human papillomavirus types associated with cervical cancer. *N Engl J Med* 2003; **348**: 518–527.
8. Frazer I. Vaccines for papillomavirus infection. *Virus Res* 2002; **89**: 271–274.
9. Syrjänen K, Syrjänen S, Lamberg M *et al.* Morphological and immunohistochemical evidence suggesting human papillomavirus (HPV) involvement in oral squamous cell carcinogenesis.

Int J Oral Surg 1983; **12**: 418–424.

10. Gillison ML, Koch WM, Capone RB *et al*. Evidence for a causal association between human papillomavirus and a subset of head and neck cancers. *J Natl Cancer Inst* 2000; **92**: 709–720.

11. Kreimer AR, Clifford GM, Boyle P, Franceschi S. Human papillomavirus types in head and neck squamous cell carcinomas worldwide: a systematic review. *Cancer Epidemiol Biomarkers Prev* 2005; **14**: 467–475.

12. Hobbs CG, Sterne JA, Bailey M *et al*. Human papillomavirus and head and neck cancer: a systematic review and meta-analysis. *Clin Otolaryngol* 2006; **31**: 259–266.

13. Zhou J, Sun XY, Stenzel DJ *et al*. Expression of vaccinia recombinant HPV 16 L1 and L2 ORF proteins in epithelial cells is sufficient for assembly of HPV virion-like particles. *Virology* 1991; **185**: 251–257.

14. Ghim SJ, Jenson AB, Schlegel R. HPV-1 L1 protein expressed in cos cells displays conformational epitopes found on intact virions. *Virology* 1992; **190**: 548–552.

15. Kirnbauer R, Booy F, Cheng N, Lowy DR, Schiller JT. Papillomavirus L1 major capsid protein self-assembles into virus-like particles that are highly immunogenic. *Proc Natl Acad Sci USA* 1992; **89**: 12180–12184.

16. Rose RC, Bonnez W, Reichman RC, Garcea RL. Expression of human papillomavirus type 11 L1 protein in insect cells: *in vivo* and *in vitro* assembly of virus like particles. *J Virol* 1993; **67**: 1936–1944.

17. Kirnbauer R, Taub J, Greenstone H *et al*. Efficient self-assembly of human papillomavirus type 16 L1 and L1-L2 into virus-like particles. *J Virol* 1993; **67**: 6929–6936.

18. Osada T, Clay TM, Woo CY, Morse MA, Lyerly HK. Dendritic cell-based immunotherapy. *Int Rev Immunol* 2006; **25**: 377–413.

19. Wang Z, Hu Q, Han W *et al*. Effect of dendritic cell vaccine against a tongue squamous cell cancer cell line (Tca8113) *in vivo* and *in vitro*. *Int J Oral Maxillofac Surg* 2006; **35**: 544–550.

20. Jeong HS, Lee H, Ko Y, Son YI. Vaccinations with dendritic cells primed with apoptotic tumor cells can elicit preventive antitumor immunity in a poorly immunogenic animal model of squamous cell carcinoma. *Laryngoscope* 2007; **117**: 1588–1593.

21. Epstein MA, Achong BG, Barr YM. Virus particles in cultured lymphoblasts from Burkitt's lymphoma. *Lancet* 1964; **15**: 702–703.

22. Henle G, Henle W, Diehl V. Relations of Burkitt's tumour-associated herpes-type virus to infectious mononucleosis. *Proc Natl Acad Sci USA* 1968; **59**: 94–101.

23. Kieff ED, Rickenson AB. Epstein–Barr virus and its replication. In: Knipe DM, Howley PM. (eds) *Field's Virology*, 5th edn. Philadelphia, PA: Lippincott Williams and Wilkins, 2007; 2603–2654.

24. Henle G, Henle W. Sereoepidemiology of the virus. In: Epstein MA, Achong BG. (eds) *The Epstein–Barr Virus*. Berlin: Springer, 1979; 297–320.

25. Sixbey JW, Nedrud JG, Raab-Traub N, Hanes RA, Pagano JS. Epstein–Barr virus replication in oropharyngeal epithelial cells. *N Engl J Med* 1984; **310**: 1225–1230.

26. Jeannel D, Bouvier G, Huber A. Nasopharyngeal carcinoma, an epidemiological approach to carcinogenesis. *Cancer Surv* 1999; **33**: 125–155.

27. Raab-Traub N, Flyn K. the structure of the termini of the Epstein–Barr virus as a marker of clonal cellular proliferation. *Cell* 1986; **47**: 883–889.

28. Khanna R, Busson P, Burrows SR *et al*. Molecular characterization of antigen-processing function in nasopharyngeal carcinoma (NPC): evidence for efficient presentation of Epstein–Barr virus cytotoxic T-cell epitopes by NPC cells. *Cancer Res* 1998; **58**: 310–314.

29. Lee SP, Constandinou CM, Thomas WA *et al*. Antigen presenting phenotype of Hodgkin–Reed–Sternberg cells: analysis of the HLA class I processing pathway and the effects of interleukin-10 on Epstein–Barr virus-specific cytotoxic T-cell recognition. *Blood* 1998; **92**: 1020–1030.

30. Straathof KC, Bollard CM, Popat U *et al*. Treatment of nasopharyngeal carcinoma with Epstein–Barr virus-specific T lymphocytes. *Blood* 2005; **105**: 1898–1904.

31. Comoli P, Pedrazzoli P, Maccario R *et al*. Cell therapy of stage IV nasopharyngeal carcinoma with autologous Epstein–Barr virus-targeted cytotoxic T lymphocytes. *J Clin Oncol* 2005; **23**: 8942–8949.

Judith A. Christian Matthew Griffin
Patrick J. Bradley

9

Chemoradiotherapy for head and neck cancer

Squamous cell carcinoma of the head and neck (HNSCC) accounts for 6% of all malignancies, and is the sixth most common cancer world-wide. Thus, the annual incidence world-wide translates into 644,000 new patients, with 352,000 dying from the disease. In Europe alone, there are 95,000 new cases of HNSCC each year, and half of these patients will die from their disease.[1] The most common sites of disease are the oral cavity, pharynx, larynx and, to a lesser extent, the nasopharynx.

Radiotherapy and surgery are the main therapeutic modalities, although there is an increasing role for chemotherapy to be added to radiotherapy as primary treatment. The choice of treatment modality depends upon the primary site, clinical stage, and resectability of the tumours. Indicators of survival include stage of disease and performance status: 5-year recurrence-free survival ranges from 91% for stage I disease to 4% for stage IVc disease.[2] Nearly two-thirds of patients present initially with advanced disease. Most failures occur within the first 2 years of treatment and around 20% of patients develop a second primary cancer in the head and neck.[3]

In the late 20th century, surgery with postoperative radiotherapy was accepted as the gold standard for advanced head and neck cancer, although

Judith A. Christian MRCP FRCR MD (for correspondence)
Consultant Clinical Oncologist, Department of Oncology, Nottingham University Hospitals, City Hospital Campus, Nottingham NG5 1PB, UK
E-mail: judith.christian@nuh.nhs.uk

Matthew Griffin MRCP FRCR
Specialist Registrar in Oncology, Department of Oncology, Nottingham University Hospitals, City Hospital Campus, Nottingham NG5 1PB, UK

Patrick J. Bradley MBA FRCS
Professor and Consultant in Head and Neck Oncologic Surgery, Department of Otolaryngology, Nottingham University Hospitals, Queen's Medical Centre Campus, Nottingham NG7 2UH, UK

many have claimed comparable results with radiation alone.[4] The VA Laryngeal Cancer Study, first published in 1991,[5] in particular stimulated head and neck oncologists to re-evaluate treatment algorithms, as the feasibility of avoiding total laryngectomy in selected patients with advanced laryngeal cancer was highlighted. A meta-analysis of 63 trials of locoregional treatment with or without chemotherapy demonstrated a survival benefit of only 4% in favour of chemotherapy of any kind.[6] An update of this meta-analysis, including an additional 24 trials showed that most of the benefit resulted from the use of chemotherapy concomitantly with radiotherapy with a 19% reduction in the risk of death and an overall 8% improvement in 5-year survival ($P < 0.0001$).[7]

In clinical practice, it is agreed that primary surgery with or without neck dissection is the treatment of choice for oral cavity, nasal cavity/sinuses, and temporal bone HNSCC tumours. Tumours located in the nasopharynx, uncommon in the UK and Europe, are treated by concomitant chemo-radiotherapy (CRT). Thus the larynx, oro- and hypo-pharynx, which are 'relatively common' sites of tumour have been considered as a group, and are currently the sites to which oncologists and surgeons discuss the role of 'organ preservation' treatment strategies. Currently, after examination and biopsy confirmation of squamous cell carcinoma, patients are staged by modern techniques, which include computed tomography (CT) and/or magnetic resonance imaging (MRI). The imaging literature distinguishing T4a (resectable) from T4b (unresectable) includes the following – carotid artery encasement, pre-vertebral fascia involvement, mediastinal infiltration, tracheal and oesophageal extension, laryngeal cartilage penetration, dural spread, bone infiltration, perineural involvement and brachial plexus invasion.[8] In a review of resected T4a and T4b oral cavity cancers, treated similarly with free-flap reconstruction and adjuvant radiotherapy or concomitant CRT, there was no statistical difference observed in the 5-year local control, neck control, disease-free survival, and overall survival rates between T4a and T4b groups.[9] Furthermore, radiological imaging has allowed for tumour volumes to be calculated, summating the primary and the nodal metastatic disease, and volumes greater than 40 ml are unlikely to respond to radiotherapy with or without chemotherapy predictably,[10] and these patients should probably be offered surgery with postoperative radiotherapy.

Thus, there are a number of clinical scenarios for which a patient's treatment and likely outcomes or survival requires clinical discussion at the multidisciplinary team meeting:

1. Patients with disease considered inoperable/unresectable and possibly incurable, when the staging process has been completed. What is the best treatment? For example, laryngeal cartilage involvement – surgery or chemoradiotherapy?

2. Patients whose tumour has been considered resectable, but the resection margins are pathologically positive, with evidence of perineural or perivascular spread. For example, T3/T4 oropharyngeal or hypopharyngeal cancer? Adjuvant radiotherapy with or without chemotherapy or primary chemoradiotherapy in future cases?

3. Patients whose tumour is considered operable, but are reluctant to consider the 'surgical morbidity' and opt for concomitant CRT, who then return with persistent locoregional disease. Has the opportunity for cure been missed? What is the surgical morbidity likely to be now?

4. Patients whose co-morbidity is such that they are unable, or are unwilling, to accept the risks of surgery, yet their tumours are considered 'curable'. For example, extensive cardiorespiratory disease?

5. Patients who present with evidence of distant metastases, but who have significant symptoms from the locoregional disease.

6. Patients who after treatment, surgery or radiotherapy with or without chemotherapy present with persistent or recurrent disease at the primary site, the regional site or locoregionally. What are the current options for treatment?

Thus, the ideal treatment for patients with advanced head and neck cancer remains unclear and must be individualised to their needs.[4] When the disease is locally advanced but resectable, surgery may result in altered functions affecting speech, swallowing and aesthetic deformity. Alternatively, both radiotherapy and chemotherapy are associated with substantial toxicity, the most common being mucositis and may equally have a major effect on a patient's quality-of-life. It is agreed that the most important issue to patients when diagnosed with a HNSCC is always survival;[11] however, when this expectation has been realised, be it in the short term, then the morbidity of the curative treatment may be questioned and complained of (e.g. shortness of breath, difficulty swallowing and change in voice).

Over the past two decades, many advances have been made not only with surgical management (free-flap reconstruction, endoscopic laser technology and partial organ surgery) but also radiotherapy, chemotherapy and biological targeted therapy. This chapter will introduce and explain the developments that have been made recently and discuss the indications and decisions that need to be considered in the treatment of advanced head and neck cancer.

CHEMORADIOTHERAPY AND ORGAN PRESERVATION

Although radiotherapy has been established as a primary treatment for carcinoma of the head and neck for many years, it is only recently that concomitant CRT has emerged as a definitive up-front treatment option for patients with resectable disease and thus has produced an attractive alternative to initial surgery. The rationale for the use of concomitant CRT is based upon the radiosensitising effects of the chemotherapy agent(s). Although concomitant CRT was originally developed for patients with inoperable disease, it has progressively become the dominant treatment modality in many centres due to the organ preservation and excellent reported local control rates. No randomised trial has, to any satisfactory extent, compared concomitant CRT with surgery and such a trial is unlikely to occur.

As discussed above, the initial Pignon et al.[6] meta-analysis showed a likely survival benefit of 8% at 5 years; however, many of these were small, underpowered trials and more recent trials have suggested a considerably greater survival benefit with an absolute risk reduction of death of 14–25% (between 4 and 7 patients need to be treated to save one life).[12–14] Phase 2 studies of concomitant CRT, which admittedly need to be viewed with some caution due to local bias, frequently show long-term survival rates of 60–70% for patients with locally advanced disease. However, a 2006 review showed that concomitant CRT benefits decrease with increasing age. Patients aged over 71 years did not benefit from concomitant CRT – the increasing risk of death from other causes with age may explain this to some extent.[15] Furthermore, the associated additional toxicity of chemotherapy requires that patients being considered for concomitant CRT fulfil the following criteria: (i) age < 70 years; (ii) good performance status (WHO PS 0 or 1); and (iii) adequate renal function (creatinine clearance > 60 ml/min).

The sensitising effect of systemic chemotherapy is not selective for tumour cells: hence, clinical trials have consistently reported an increase in the incidence of toxic normal tissue effects with the use of concomitant CRT in HNSCC, particularly in regard to grade 3 and 4 mucositis and dermatitis.[16]

When selecting patients for concomitant CRT, long-term sequelae and their effects on quality-of-life need serious consideration. Sensorineural hearing loss develops in about one-third of patients after curative radiation doses and can be progressive.[17] Cisplatin chemotherapy adds to this ototoxicity and could potentiate the propensity for deafness. The potential for aspiration following chemoradiotherapy is probably under-reported in the literature and has been found to develop in up to 59% of patients undergoing chemoradiotherapy.[18] This has important implications for the nutrition of the patient undergoing chemoradiotherapy and may necessitate prolonged dependence upon a gastrostomy feeding tube.

A prospective study assessing quality-of-life parameters in patients undergoing concomitant CRT for locally advanced head and neck cancer found that acute end of treatment toxicities were severe with declines in virtually all quality-of-life and functional domains studied.[19] Although by 12 months there was marked improvement in general functional and physical measures, up to a third of patients continued to report problems with swallowing, hoarseness, mouth pain, dry mouth, loss of taste and need for a soft diet. This re-emphasises the need for these patients to be treated in a specialist centre where adequate multidisciplinary support services are available.

CYTOTOXIC AGENTS

Cisplatin is a potent radiosensitiser and is the most studied cytotoxic agent in head and neck cancer. Evidence suggests that regimens containing cisplatin offer a 12% risk reduction over non-platinum based regimens ($P < 0.00001$), and a schedule of 100 mg/m^2 administered 3-weekly during radiotherapy is the most widely adopted regimen internationally.[20] This treatment potentially has significant toxic effects including nephrotoxicity, ototoxicity, and neurotoxicity as well as an exacerbation of local radiotherapy effects and is, therefore, suitable only for those patients of otherwise good performance status and with normal renal function. Attempts to limit the toxicity of the treatment have included administering a smaller dose of cisplatin on a weekly basis concurrently with radiotherapy, and reduced toxicity has been reported with this regimen in phase II clinical trials; as yet, there is no comparative data to support the routine use of this regimen.

For patients unable to tolerate cisplatin due to pre-existing impairment of renal function, carboplatin can be substituted. Carboplatin, a cisplatin derivative, has been studied due to its more favourable side-effect profile and relative ease of administration. The radiosensitising effects of carboplatin are not as well established as those of cisplatin although one study has shown similar efficacy.[21] No agent has yet been shown to be superior to cisplatin in terms of survival benefit. In recent years, there has been considerable interest in the taxanes as potent radiosensitisers and a phase II study using weekly docetaxel with standard radiotherapy has reported a 3-year overall survival of 47% (95% CI, 39–68%).[22] The main side-effects were grade 3 or 4 mucositis (84%) and dermatitis (53%), with relatively infrequent haematological toxic effects (5% rate of grade 3 or 4 neutropenia). Paclitaxel administered weekly with concurrent radiotherapy produced manageable side-effects in phase II studies with response rates of up to 65% and 2-year survival of 46% reported.[23]

Combination chemotherapy schedules have undergone numerous small phase II trials. 5-fluorouracil (5-FU) is well established as a radiosensitiser and many studies have explored the efficacy of combining cisplatin and 5-FU concurrently with radiotherapy in the treatment of HNSCC, and improved locoregional control rates and trends towards improved survival have been reported.[24 26] The overlapping toxicity of oral mucositis from the 5-FU makes this intuitively a less desirable schedule, although it remains fairly widely used.

Progressively, however, it will be the newer taxane drugs which will feature in chemoradiotherapy drug trial combinations. One multicentre randomised phase II trial compared the use of concomitant CRT using either cisplatin+5-FU, cisplatin+paclitaxel or 5-FU+hydroxyurea.[27] Both the cisplatin+paclitaxel and the 5-FU+hydroxyurea combinations produced superior 2-year overall survival when compared to cisplatin+5-FU. Data from a pathological series assessing induction chemotherapy in HNSCC showed that a complete pathological response was found at 89% of biopsy proven primary sites when a taxane+cisplatin+5-FU drug combination was used compared to the 25–50% complete response rate previously reported in other pathological series using a cisplatin+5-FU only combination.[28] The results of these studies suggest that multi-drug combinations may provide superior outcomes in the treatment of head and neck cancers and that taxanes may be an important component of these regimens. No randomised trial has yet adequately compared these combinations with single-agent cisplatin chemoradiotherapy and thus it remains the current standard of care.

IMPROVING RADIOTHERAPY SCHEDULES

Attempts to improve outcomes for patients with locally advanced HNSCC have also focused upon modification of radiotherapy fractionation schedules.[29] Traditionally, conventional radiotherapy has consisted of once daily treatment delivering 2 Gy per day, 5 days per week to a total dose of 70 Gy over 7 weeks. Based on radiobiological principles, two altered fractionation schedules have been studied – hyperfractionation and accelerated fractionation:

1. **Hyperfractionation** delivers a higher total dose over the same 7-week treatment period using multiple smaller fractions of radiotherapy per day. The lower dose per fraction results in preferential sparing of late-responding tissues thus reducing the incidence of late normal-tissue effects.

2. **Accelerated fractionation** delivers the same total dose over a shorter overall treatment time and is aimed at overcoming treatment failures caused by tumour-cell repopulation during longer courses of treatment.

The Radiation Therapy Oncology Group (RTOG) carried out a phase III study comparing four fractionation schedules – (i) conventional fractionation; (ii) hyperfractionation (1.2 Gy twice daily to a total dose of 81.6 Gy); (iii) accelerated radiotherapy with a concomitant boost (1.8 Gy daily, 5 days per week, with a second fraction of 1.5 Gy daily during the final 12 days to a total dose of 72 Gy); and (iv) 1.6 Gy given twice daily with a 2-week break to deliver a total dose of 67.2 Gy.[30] Improved local control was seen both in patients treated with hyperfractionated radiotherapy and those treated with the accelerated schedule with concomitant boost, although no difference in overall survival was seen. A meta-analysis of 15 trials including over 6500 patients treated with either hyperfractionated or accelerated radiotherapy schedules has shown a significant survival benefit of 3.4% at 5 years in favour of altered fractionation regimens.[31] The benefit was significantly higher with hyperfractionated radiotherapy (8% at 5 years) than with accelerated radiotherapy (2% without total dose reduction, 1.7% with total dose reduction at 5 years; $P = 0.02$). The radiotherapy dose-fractionation studies have mostly been carried out in the setting of radiotherapy as single modality treatment. Attempts at combining altered fractionation schedules with chemotherapy in small studies have often shown high levels of toxicity and poor patient tolerance. The added value of altered radiotherapy dose-fractionation is not yet known in the context of concomitant CRT and the results of two randomised trials are awaited to address this issue.[29]

POSTOPERATIVE CHEMORADIATION FOR HIGH-RISK CANCERS

Predictors of recurrence after surgical resection include involved margins of resection, extranodal/extracapsular spread, perineural invasion, and the presence of two or more involved regional lymph nodes. Locoregional failures remain a dominant problem, and adjuvant (postoperative) radiotherapy was known to decrease local failure rates – indeed, since the 1980s, was considered to also increase survival. Even with adjuvant radiotherapy, in the presence of high-risk features, the risk of local recurrence (27–62%), distant metastases (18–21%), and death (5-year survival rate 27–34%) remains unsatisfactory.[32] Thus postoperative (adjuvant) chemoradiotherapy offered an approach that could enhance local control with the addition of radiosensitising agents. Recently, two multicentric randomised trials, the RTOG 9501[33] and the EORTC 22931,[34] produced level I evidence of a clear benefit for adjuvant chemoradiotherapy at the cost of increase in acute toxicities. Although only the EORTC trial showed a significant survival advantage for chemoradiotherapy, the RTOG trial trend was in the same direction and showed a significant increase in progression-free survival. In both trials, there was an increase in acute grade III and IV toxicities in the combined arm, including toxic deaths. At present, for patients without high-risk features, the evidence of benefit of chemoradiotherapy over radiation alone is less clear with no randomised trials addressing this question. One of the results, which needs to be recognised, is that the locoregional failure rate remains unsatisfactorily high at 30%. The optimal time to start adjuvant treatment post-surgery has not been studied sufficiently. Limited evidence and clinical experience with the time needed for patients to recover suggests that it should be within 4–6 weeks of surgery.

Many questions regarding the optimisation of adjuvant treatments remain unanswered, especially with respect to improvement of patient compliance, integration of novel drugs targeting both locoregional and systemic control, and modulation of treatment intensity according to risk levels.[35]

THE ROLE OF ADJUVANT LYMPH NODE DISSECTION

When surgery is chosen as the primary treatment modality for HNSCC, standard practice dictates that neck dissection should be performed at the time of initial resection in those patients at risk of, or who are known to have, node positive disease. However, following the development of concomitant CRT, the role of neck dissection has become somewhat controversial.[36] General consensus exists that neck dissection is unnecessary in those patients with N1 disease who have complete clinical/radiological response following concomitant CRT. For those with N2/3 disease, advocates of adjuvant neck dissection argue that clinical and radiological complete response does not accurately correlate with pathological complete response, and that approximately 25% of patients with a clinically negative neck will have residual nodal disease confirmed after neck dissection.[37] Other investigators suggest that adjuvant neck dissection is unnecessary following concomitant CRT as it will not reduce the risk of regional recurrence or distant failure and, therefore, will not improve overall survival; morbidity, however, will be increased.[38] Furthermore, 30–40% of patients who have less than a clinical or radiological complete response in the neck have no residual tumour identified at surgery. A recent study of 154 patients undergoing chemoradiotherapy using hyperfractionated radiotherapy found that adjuvant modified neck dissection still appears to confer a disease-free survival and overall survival advantage in those patients with N2/3 disease who had a clinical complete response following chemoradiotherapy.[38] Realistically, patient choice will have a major impact on the decision for neck dissection or not. The toxicity of concomitant CRT and associated severe short-term morbidity may make patients decline any further surgical intervention, which may, from their point of view, be unnecessary as their disease has already been clinically eradicated.

IMAGING AFTER CHEMORADIATION

It is hoped that advances in imaging technology may help to differentiate further those patients who may be simply observed after completing chemoradiotherapy from those that would benefit from an adjuvant neck lymph node dissection. Fluorodeoxyglucose-positron emission tomography

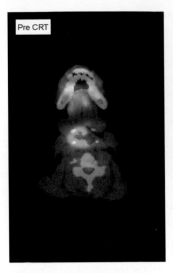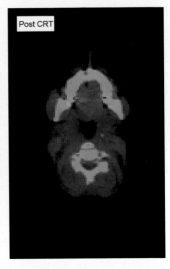

Fig. 1 A patient with a T4 N0 pharyngeal squamous cell carcinoma before and after concomitant CRT with a complete response shown on FDG-PET images.

(FDG-PET) scanning has been shown to be more accurate than CT or MRI in the post-radiotherapy setting by several studies (Fig. 1). Furthermore, there is evidence that patients who have a clinical and radiological complete response as well as a negative PET scan 12 weeks after completing chemoradiotherapy may be appropriately observed without undergoing surgery.[39–41]

A recent study to determine whether post-radiotherapy FDG-PET can predict the pathological status of residual cervical lymph nodes in patients undergoing definitive radiotherapy for HNSCC found that using a SUV_{max} of less than 3.0 as the criterion for a negative FDG-PET study, the sensitivity, specificity, positive predictive value, and negative predictive value were 100%, 84.2%, 62.5% and 100%, respectively.[42] This again supports the view that those with a negative FDG-PET study may be observed after definitive radiotherapy treatment and that a prospective clinical trial is warranted to determine if this is the case.

A CHANGING ROLE FOR INDUCTION CHEMOTHERAPY

Chemotherapy is now an established integral part of the curative treatment for HNSCC but uncertainty remains as to its optimum use in combined modality treatment. With increasingly effective local control measures, there is now a majority of patients that will fail therapy with distant metastases, presumably from micrometastatic disease, that local therapy with lower dose chemotherapy was unable to treat adequately. The rationale for using induction chemotherapy is:

- reduction in the bulk of tumour cells prior to definitive treatment – either surgery or radiotherapy

- improved drug delivery with an undisturbed blood supply

- avoidance of overlapping treatment toxicity
- early systemic treatment of micrometastatic disease.

The main drawbacks of induction treatment are the possibilities of delaying definitive treatment and of introducing tumour resistance.

The several meta-analyses evaluating the use of chemotherapy in HNSCC have shown most benefit using concomitant CRT compared with the benefit seen with induction chemotherapy followed by radiotherapy alone.[6] Within the original MACH-NC meta-analysis, a sub-analysis found that platinum-containing regimens gave a significant 5% absolute survival benefit at 5 years ($P < 0.01$) when chemotherapy was given solely as an induction regimen and not concomitant with radiotherapy.[43] However, individual studies have failed to show a survival advantage consistently, but those that do show a reduction in the incidence of distant metastases as the first site of failure.[6,44–46]

Until recently, the regimen most commonly used for induction chemotherapy was cisplatin+5-FU. This has been challenged by a newer triplet regimen of cisplatin+5-FU+taxane (paclitaxel or docetaxel), known as TPF. Two trials have compared these induction regimens followed by local treatment in stage III and IV head and neck cancer (Table 1).[47,48]

Although one of these studies is yet to report fully, the data are encouraging for a survival benefit using TPF induction chemotherapy with very reasonable toxicity profiles. As it stands, however, induction chemotherapy should still be considered experimental treatment although the above studies form an excellent basis for randomised trials comparing the best induction regimens

Table 1 Trial results of the newer triplet regimen of cisplatin+5-FU+taxane (paclitaxel or docetaxel), known as TPF

Trial	n	Induction therapy	Local therapy	Toxic deaths	Organ preserv.	Survival benefit
Hitt et al.[47]	382	PF x 3	CRT	2.1%	52%	Yes in favour of TPF
		TPF x 3	CRT	1.1%	63%	2-year OS 53.6% vs 66.5%; $P = 0.06$
		(T = paclitaxel)		(NS)	$P < 0.049$	Most benefit in unresectable disease
Remenar et al.[48]	358	PF x 4	RT/S	7.8%	Not reported	Yes in favour of TPF
EORTC 24971		TPF x 4	RT/S	3.7%	Not reported	3-year OS 23.9% vs 36.5% HR 0.71; $P = 0.0052$
TAX 323		(T = docetaxel)				

P, cisplatin; F, 5-fluorouracil; CRT, chemoradiotherapy; T, taxane; S, surgery; NS, not significant; EORTC, European Organisation for Research and Treatment of Cancer; organ preserv., organ preservation; P, probability.

followed by concomitant CRT with concomitant CRT alone. Thus, it is likely that induction chemotherapy and concomitant chemotherapy might have complementary effects on overall disease control – induction chemotherapy reducing the incidence of distant metastasis and concomitant chemotherapy improving locoregional control. However, these trials have yet to be performed.

NOVEL AGENTS IN COMBINATION WITH RADIOTHERAPY

With the current concomitant CRT treatments having essentially reached their intensification maxima, it falls upon newer therapies to improve efficacy and reduce the toxicity of head and neck cancer treatments. New anti-cancer drugs are being developed which interact with defined tumour-associated molecular targets. Drugs targeting tumour epidermal growth factor receptors (EGFRs) and their downstream signalling pathways have a compelling rationale in head and neck cancer. Overexpression of EGFR has been observed in over 80% of HNSCC.[49,50] Epidermal growth factor (EGF) stimulates the growth of several types of epithelial tissues and possesses a strong mitogenic activity that is mediated through its cell surface receptor. EGFR overexpression is associated with aggressive tumour growth and, hence, shorter relapse-free and overall survival rates.[49,50] It is, therefore, a highly significant factor in the biology of HNSCC.

Cetuximab is a monoclonal antibody which targets EGFR with a high affinity and blocks its action by stimulating receptor internalisation and degradation.

Bonner et al.[51] reported a large series of patients (n = 424) with locally advanced HNSCC who were treated with either radiotherapy alone or radiotherapy in combination with cetuximab.[51,52] The addition of cetuximab to radiotherapy significantly improved survival and locoregional control compared to radiotherapy alone. Median survival in the cetuximab arm was 49 months, almost 20 months longer than with radiotherapy alone (29.3 months; P = 0.03). Cetuximab plus radiotherapy was associated with a 26% reduction in mortality compared with radiotherapy alone (hazard ratio (HR), 0.74) and produced a 32% reduction in locoregional failure compared to radiotherapy alone (HR, 0.68). Cetuximab was well tolerated, the common side-effect being of a mild-to-moderate acneiform rash in the majority of patients. Of particular importance, it did not enhance the acute mucosal side effects of the radiotherapy, unlike other concomitant CRT agents (e.g. cisplatin). This trial paves the way for others assessing the efficacy of cetuximab and other EGFR blocking drugs in combination with concomitant CRT and provides an alternative treatment option for patients not amenable to standard cytotoxic therapy.

ADVANCES IN RADIOTHERAPY

3-D CONFORMAL RADIOTHERAPY

The radiotherapy treatment of HNSCC has made significant advances over recent years with the development of 3-D conformal radiotherapy (3D-RT).

This uses CT images within the radiotherapy planning system to define with greater accuracy the primary tumour and its associated lymph nodes. In addition, it has permitted a greater assessment of doses to surrounding normal tissues which are know to be highly sensitive to radiation (*e.g.* spinal cord, salivary glands, lens and optic chiasm). Accurate estimates of the actual dose given to both the tumour and normal tissues can be made allowing for the generation of radiotherapy plans, which reduce radiation dose to normal tissues but allow escalation of dose to the tumour. Despite these advances, 3-D radiotherapy in the head and neck region still has limitations in the shape of the dose distribution it is able to create; for example, 3-D radiotherapy often encompasses the tumour and associated lymphatics using two opposed lateral fields, which are particularly unable to avoid the radiation-sensitive parotid glands. This unavoidable irradiation of the parotid glands during 3-D radiotherapy (for mainly nasopharyngeal and oropharyngeal tumours) results in hyposalivation as a consequence of permanent damage to the parotid glands. The resultant xerostomia can significantly impair quality-of-life and is the commonest long-term side-effect of radiation treatment. Studies have repeatedly shown that xerostomia can cause oral discomfort and pain, increased dental caries and oral infection, and difficulty speaking and swallowing. This has been found to impair long-term quality-of-life significantly and can compromise nutritional intake.[52,53]

INTENSITY-MODULATED RADIOTHERAPY

Intensity-modulated radiotherapy (IMRT) is an advanced computer-optimised technology for radiation planning and delivery. It was introduced in an attempt to improve the ability of standard 3-D radiotherapy to deliver a high dose of radiation to the tumour more precisely whilst minimising the dose to the surrounding normal tissues (*e.g.* parotid glands and spinal cord) by the creation of concave dose distributions. These concave dose distributions are able to 'wrap' themselves around the target volume keeping the nearby normal structures out of the high-dose area. Parotid-sparing IMRT is becoming a key treatment approach in the management of HNSCC because of its capacity for reducing parotid radiation dose and, thereby, reducing radiotherapy-related side-effects that lead to long-term psychological and functional morbidity. A study by Braam *et al.*[54] showed that 41% of patients still complain of moderate or severe xerostomia at 5-year follow-up after 3-D radiotherapy to the head and neck. In a comparative study of 3-D radiotherapy and IMRT, Braam *et al.*[54] showed the mean stimulated parotid flow ratio 6 weeks and 6 months for a series of 56 patients treated with radiotherapy for oropharyngeal cancer to be 41% and 64% for IMRT and 11% and 18% for 3-D radiotherapy, respectively. The number of parotid flow complications 6 months after treatment was 56% for IMRT and 81% for 3-D radiotherapy ($P = 0.04$). There is also growing evidence that IMRT can very significantly reduce high-dose volumes to the mandible thus impacting on rates of osteoradionecrosis and, hence, improved osseo-integration of dental implants.[55]

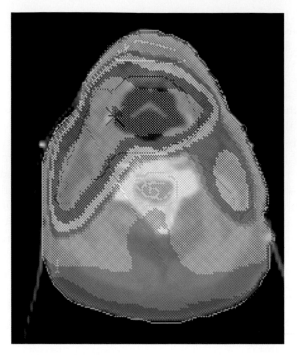

Fig. 2 A typical IMRT dose distribution.

Figure 2 shows an IMRT dose distribution for a patient undergoing radiotherapy for an oropharyngeal carcinoma, with the high-dose area (green) in a concave distribution around the spinal cord and the contralateral parotid gland removed from the high-dose volume. At the same time, there is good evidence that there is no reduction in local control with IMRT despite the smaller treatment volumes.[56,57] IMRT is, however, considerably more resource intensive, at least in the early years of a radiotherapy centre developing the technique, than standard 3-D radiotherapy in terms of physics staff-time and radiotherapy quality assurance. Hence, many centres have struggled to develop their IMRT programmes and 3-D radiotherapy remains the current UK standard for radiotherapy.

CONCLUSIONS

Concomitant CRT has established itself as a definitive therapy for locally advanced HNSCC and in the postoperative setting due to the organ preservation and high levels of local control achieved. It will continue to evolve as new cytotoxic drugs (such as the taxanes) are introduced and with the progressive use of EGFR-targeted therapies, which are likely to reduce the toxicity of treatment. In the future, the use of FDG-PET imaging may help in decision-making regarding which patients require further surgery. As overall survival rates improve, clear outcome measures will be crucial in determining which treatments are superior at providing both cure and a good quality-of-life.

Key points for clinical practice

- The treatment of head and neck squamous cell carcinoma (HNSCC) has evolved considerably over the last two decades with increasing importance being placed on organ preservation and the patient's long-term quality of life after treatment.

- The use of platinum-based concomitant chemoradiotherapy gives at least an 8% improvement in 5-year survival when compared to radiotherapy alone. The incidence of toxic effects, particularly mucositis and dermatitis, is significantly increased.

- Cisplatin chemotherapy administered concurrently with radiotherapy is the most studied and the most utilised concomitant CRT regimen. There is increasing evidence of efficacy of multi-agent regimens in the concurrent setting (particularly using taxane drugs) but none has yet been shown to be superior to cisplatin alone.

- Most radiotherapy in the UK is delivered at 2 Gy per fraction per day. As a single-modality treatment, hyperfractionated radiotherapy produces a survival benefit of similar magnitude to the addition of chemotherapy to conventionally fractionated radiotherapy. The role of chemotherapy when used with alternative radiotherapy fractionation schedules remains to be determined.

- Postoperative chemoradiotherapy with high-dose cisplatin (100 mg/m^2 on days 1, 22, 43 of radiotherapy) and radiation doses of at least 60–66 Gy is more effective than adjuvant radiation alone in the post-operative setting for patients with high-risk of developing a recurrence. The patients who benefit most from this approach are those with positive surgical margins and/or nodal extracapsular spread.

- There is controversy surrounding the role of adjuvant neck dissection for patients with N2 and N3 disease after concomitant chemoradiotherapy. Fluorodeoxyglucose-positron emission tomography imaging is more accurate than either computed tomography or magnetic resonance imaging following treatment and may help to differentiate between those patients requiring adjuvant neck dissection and those that do not.

- Induction chemotherapy using taxane+cisplatin-based chemotherapy may improve overall survival if followed by concomitant CRT. Induction chemotherapy is still considered experimental and further data required before it becomes standard management.

- Epidermal growth factor receptors (EGFRs) are overexpressed in HNSCC and are associated with poor prognosis. The monoclonal antibody cetuximab blocks EGFR and has been found to improve median survival and locoregional control when added to radiotherapy compared to radiotherapy alone.

- Intensity modulated radiotherapy is a new method of radiotherapy treatment planning and delivery, which allows the treatment of concave tumour volumes. This is predominantly used in HNSCC to allow parotid-sparing radiotherapy.

References

1. Parkin DM, Bray F, Ferlay J, Pisani P. Global cancer statistics, 2002. *CA Cancer J Clin* 2005; **55**: 74–108.
2. Iro H, Waldfahrer F. Evaluation of the newly updated TNM classification of head and neck carcinoma with data from 3247 patients. *Cancer* 1998; **83**: 2201–2207.
3. Verschuur HP, Irish JC, O'Sullivan B, Goh C, Gullane PJ, Pintilie M. A matched control study of treatment outcome in young patients with squamous cell carcinoma of the head and neck. *Laryngoscope* 1999; **109**: 249–258.
4. Gleich LL, Collins CM, Gartside PS *et al*. Therapeutic decision making in stages III and IV head and neck squamous cell carcinoma. *Arch Otolaryngol Head Neck Surg* 2003; **129**: 26–35.
5. The Department of Veterans Affairs Laryngeal Cancer Study Group. Induction chemotherapy plus radiation compared with surgery plus radiation in patients with advanced laryngeal cancer. *N Engl J Med* 1991; **324**: 1685–1690.
6. Pignon JP, Bourhis J, Domenge C, Designe L. Chemotherapy added to locoregional treatment for head and neck squamous-cell carcinoma: three meta-analyses of updated individual data. MACH-NC Collaborative Group. Meta-Analysis of Chemotherapy on Head and Neck Cancer. *Lancet* 2000; **355**: 949–955.
7. Pignon JP, Baujat B, Bourhis J. Individual patient data meta-analyses in head and neck carcinoma: what have we learnt? *Cancer Radiother* 2005; **9**: 31–36.
8. Yousem DM, Gad K, Tufano RP. Resectability issues with head and neck cancer. *AJNR Am J Neuroradiol* 2006; **27**: 2024–2036.
9. Liao CT, Chang JT, Wang HM *et al*. Surgical outcome of T4a and resected T4b oral cavity cancer. *Cancer* 2006; **107**: 337–344.
10. Chen SW, Yang SN, Liang JA, Tsai MH, Shiau AC, Lin FJ. Value of computed tomography-based tumor volume as a predictor of outcomes in hypopharyngeal cancer after treatment with definitive radiotherapy. *Laryngoscope* 2006; **116**: 2012–2017.
11. List MA, Stracks J, Colangelo L *et al*. How do head and neck cancer patients prioritize treatment outcomes before initiating treatment? *J Clin Oncol* 2000; **18**: 877–884.
12. Seiwert TY, Cohen EE. State-of-the-art management of locally advanced head and neck cancer. *Br J Cancer* 2005; **92**: 1341–1348.
13. Adelstein DJ, Li Y, Adams GL *et al*. An intergroup phase III comparison of standard radiation therapy and two schedules of concurrent chemoradiotherapy in patients with unresectable squamous cell head and neck cancer. *J Clin Oncol* 2003; **21**: 92–98.
14. Brizel DM, Albers ME, Fisher SR *et al*. Hyperfractionated irradiation with or without concurrent chemotherapy for locally advanced head and neck cancer. *N Engl J Med* 1998; **338**: 1798–1804.
15. Bourhis J, Le Maitre A, Pignon JP *et al*. Impact of age on treatment effect in locally advanced head and neck cancer (HNC): Two individual patient data meta-analyses. *J Clin Oncol* 2006; **24 (Suppl)**: 18S, abstract 5501.
16. Seiwert TY, Salama JK, Vokes EE. The chemoradiation paradigm in head and neck cancer. *Nat Clin Pract Oncol* 2007; **4**: 156–171.
17. Grau C, Overgaard J. Postirradiation sensorineural hearing loss: a common but ignored late radiation complication. *Int J Radiat Oncol Biol Phys* 1996; **36**: 515–517.
18. Nguyen NP, Frank C, Moltz CC *et al*. Aspiration rate following chemoradiation for head and neck cancer: an underreported occurrence. *Radiother Oncol* 2006; **80**: 302–306.
19. List MA, Siston A, Haraf D *et al*. Quality of life and performance in advanced head and neck cancer patients on concomitant chemoradiotherapy: a prospective examination. *J Clin Oncol* 1999; **17**: 1020–1028.
20. Browman GP, Hodson DI, Mackenzie RJ, Bestic N, Zuraw L. Choosing a concomitant chemotherapy and radiotherapy regimen for squamous cell head and neck cancer: a systematic review of the published literature with subgroup analysis. *Head Neck* 2001; **23**: 579–589.
21. Jeremic B, Shibamoto Y, Stanisavljevic B, Milojevic L, Milicic B, Nikolic N. Radiation therapy alone or with concurrent low-dose daily either cisplatin or carboplatin in locally advanced unresectable squamous cell carcinoma of the head and neck: a prospective randomized trial. *Radiother Oncol* 1997; **43**: 29–37.
22. Calais G, Bardet E, Sire C *et al*. Radiotherapy with concomitant weekly docetaxel for

Stages III/IV oropharynx carcinoma. Results of the 98-02 GORTEC Phase II trial. *Int J Radiat Oncol Biol Phys* 2004; **58**: 161–166.

23. Lovey J, Koronczay K, Remenar E, Csuka O, Nemeth G. Radiotherapy and concurrent low-dose paclitaxel in locally advanced head and neck cancer. *Radiother Oncol* 2003; **68**: 171–174.

24. Adelstein DJ, Saxton JP, Rybicki LA *et al.* Multiagent concurrent chemoradiotherapy for locoregionally advanced squamous cell head and neck cancer: mature results from a single institution. *J Clin Oncol* 2006; **24**: 1064–1071.

25. Brizel DM, Albers ME, Fisher SR *et al.* Hyperfractionated irradiation with or without concurrent chemotherapy for locally advanced head and neck cancer. *N Engl J Med* 1998; **338**: 1798–1804.

26. Taylor SG, Murthy AK, Vannetzel JM *et al.* Randomized comparison of neoadjuvant cisplatin and fluorouracil infusion followed by radiation versus concomitant treatment in advanced head and neck cancer. *J Clin Oncol* 1994; **12**: 385–395.

27. Garden AS, Harris J, Vokes EE *et al.* Preliminary results of Radiation Therapy Oncology Group 97-03: a randomized phase II trial of concurrent radiation and chemotherapy for advanced squamous cell carcinomas of the head and neck. *J Clin Oncol* 2004; **22**: 2856–2864.

28. Haddad R, Tishler R, Wirth L *et al.* Rate of pathologic complete responses to docetaxel, cisplatin, and fluorouracil induction chemotherapy in patients with squamous cell carcinoma of the head and neck. *Arch Otolaryngol Head Neck Surg* 2006; **132**: 678–681.

29. Ang KK. Concurrent radiation chemotherapy for locally advanced head and neck carcinoma: are we addressing burning subjects? *J Clin Oncol* 2004; **22**: 4657–4659

30. Fu KK, Pajak TF, Trotti A *et al.* A Radiation Therapy Oncology Group (RTOG) phase III randomized study to compare hyperfractionation and two variants of accelerated fractionation to standard fractionation radiotherapy for head and neck squamous cell carcinomas: first report of RTOG 9003. *Int J Radiat Oncol Biol Phys* 2000; **48**: 7–16.

31. Bourhis J, Overgaard J, Audry H *et al.* Hyperfractionated or accelerated radiotherapy in head and neck cancer: a meta-analysis. *Lancet* 2006; **368**: 843–854.

32. Cooper JS, Pajak TF, Forastiere A *et al.* Precisely defining high-risk operable head and neck tumors based on RTOG #85-03 and #88-24: targets for postoperative radiochemotherapy? *Head Neck* 1998; **20**: 588–594.

33. Cooper JS, Pajak TF, Forastiere AA *et al.* Postoperative concurrent radiotherapy and chemotherapy for high-risk squamous-cell carcinoma of the head and neck. *N Engl J Med* 2004; **350**: 1937–1944.

34. Bernier J, Domenge C, Ozsahin M *et al.* Postoperative irradiation with or without concomitant chemotherapy for locally advanced head and neck cancer. *N Engl J Med* 2004; **350**: 1945–1952.

35. Bernier J, Vermorken JB, Koch WM. Adjuvant therapy in patients with resected poor-risk head and neck cancer. *J Clin Oncol* 2006; **24**: 2629–2635.

36. McHam SA, Adelstein DJ, Rybicki LA *et al.* Who merits a neck dissection after definitive chemoradiotherapy for N2–N3 squamous cell head and neck cancer? *Head Neck* 2003; **25**: 791–798.

37. Brizel DM, Esclamado R. Concurrent chemoradiotherapy for locally advanced, nonmetastatic, squamous carcinoma of the head and neck: consensus, controversy, and conundrum. *J Clin Oncol* 2006; **24**: 2612–2617.

38. Brizel DM, Prosnitz RG, Hunter S *et al.* Necessity for adjuvant neck dissection in setting of concurrent chemoradiation for advanced head-and-neck cancer. *Int J Radiat Oncol Biol Phys* 2004; **58**: 1418–1423.

39. Yao M, Smith RB, Graham MM *et al.* The role of FDG PET in management of neck metastasis from head-and-neck cancer after definitive radiation treatment. *Int J Radiat Oncol Biol Phys* 2005; **63**: 991–999.

40. Farber LA, Benard F, Machtay M *et al.* Detection of recurrent head and neck squamous cell carcinomas after radiation therapy with 2-^{18}F-fluoro-2-deoxy-D-glucose positron emission tomography. *Laryngoscope* 1999; **109**: 970–975.

41. Kubota K, Yokoyama J, Yamaguchi K *et al.* FDG-PET delayed imaging for the detection of head and neck cancer recurrence after radio-chemotherapy: comparison with MRI/CT. *Eur J Nucl Med Mol Imaging* 2004; **31**: 590–595.

42. Yao M, Luo P, Hoffman HT et al. Pathology and FDG PET correlation of residual lymph nodes in head and neck cancer after radiation treatment. Am J Clin Oncol 2007; 30: 264–270.

43. Monnerat C, Faivre S, Temam S, Bourhis J, Raymond E. End points for new agents in induction chemotherapy for locally advanced head and neck cancers. Ann Oncol 2002; 13: 995–1006.

44. Adjuvant chemotherapy for advanced head and neck squamous carcinoma. Final report of the Head and Neck Contracts Program. Cancer 1987; 60: 301–311.

45. Paccagnella A, Orlando A, Marchiori C et al. Phase III trial of initial chemotherapy in stage III or IV head and neck cancers: a study by the Gruppo di Studio sui Tumori della Testa e del Collo. J Natl Cancer Inst 1994; 86: 265–272.

46. Lefebvre JL, Chevalier D, Luboinski B, Kirkpatrick A, Collette L, Sahmoud T. Larynx preservation in pyriform sinus cancer: preliminary results of a European Organization for Research and Treatment of Cancer phase III trial. EORTC Head and Neck Cancer Cooperative Group. J Natl Cancer Inst 1996; 88: 890–899.

47. Hitt R, Lopez-Pousa A, Martinez-Trufero J et al. Phase III study comparing cisplatin plus fluorouracil to paclitaxel, cisplatin, and fluorouracil induction chemotherapy followed by chemoradiotherapy in locally advanced head and neck cancer. J Clin Oncol 2005; 23: 8636–8645.

48. Remenar E, van Herpen C, Germa Lluch J et al. A randomized phase III multicenter trial of neoadjuvant docetaxel (Taxotere) plus cisplatin plus 5-fluorouracil (TPF) versus neoadjuvant cisplatin plus 5-fluorouracil (PF) in patients with locally advanced unresectable squamous cell carcinoma of the head and neck (SCCHN): final analysis of EORTC protocol 24971. J Clin Oncol 2006; 24 (Suppl): 18S, abstract, 5516.

49. Santini J, Formento JL, Francoual M et al. Characterization, quantification, and potential clinical value of the epidermal growth factor receptor in head and neck squamous cell carcinomas. Head Neck 1991; 13: 132–139.

50. Grandis JR, Melhem MF, Gooding WE et al. Levels of TGF-alpha and EGFR protein in head and neck squamous cell carcinoma and patient survival. J Natl Cancer Inst 1998; 90: 824–832.

51. Bonner JA, Harari PM, Giralt J et al. Radiotherapy plus cetuximab for squamous-cell carcinoma of the head and neck. N Engl J Med 2006; 354: 567–578.

52. Epstein JB, Robertson M, Emerton S, Phillips N, Stevenson-Moore P. Quality of life and oral function in patients treated with radiation therapy for head and neck cancer. Head Neck 2001; 23: 389–398.

53. Chambers MS, Garden AS, Kies MS, Martin JW. Radiation-induced xerostomia in patients with head and neck cancer: pathogenesis, impact on quality of life, and management. Head Neck 2004; 26: 796–807.

54. Braam PM, Roesink JM, Raaijmakers CP, Busschers WB, Terhaard CH. Quality of life and salivary output in patients with head-and-neck cancer five years after radiotherapy. Radiat Oncol 2007; 2: 3.

55. Studer G, Studer SP, Zwahlen RA et al. Osteoradionecrosis of the mandible: minimized risk profile following intensity-modulated radiation therapy (IMRT). Strahlenther Onkol 2006; 182: 283–288.

56. Milano MT, Vokes EE, Kao J et al. Intensity-modulated radiation therapy in advanced head and neck patients treated with intensive chemoradiotherapy: preliminary experience and future directions. Int J Oncol 2006; 28: 1141–1151.

57. Yao M, Dornfeld KJ, Buatti JM et al. Intensity-modulated radiation treatment for head-and-neck squamous cell carcinoma – the University of Iowa experience. Int J Radiat Oncol Biol Phys 2005; 63: 410–421.

Anshul Sama Nick S. Jones

10

Image-guided surgery in paranasal sinus and skull base surgery

In 1996, the International Society for Computer-Aided Surgery (ISCAS) defined the scope of computer-aided surgery (CAS) as encompassing 'all fields within surgery, as well as biomedical imaging and instrumentation, and digital technology employed as adjunct to imaging in diagnosis, therapeutics, and surgery'.[1] CAS, therefore, includes surgical navigation, virtual reality, computer-aided image review, stereotactic surgery, robotic surgery, telemedicine, computer-aided tumour modelling and many other applications. Within the field of otorhinolaryngology, head and neck surgery, CAS has had its major impact in the field of endoscopic sinus surgery (ESS) in the form of intra operative surgical navigation commonly termed 'image-guided surgery' (IGS). Although this technology has been in applied for over two decades, it is only in the last decade that its usage has become more extensive. Instrumental in this rise has been significant advancements in technology. This article reviews the most recent advances and possible associated limitations.

ACCURACY

Accuracy is fundamentally the most important issue in image-guided surgery. If it were perfect then it would be possible to operate from the image-guided system alone. In the past, it has been argued that an accuracy of 2–3 mm should be achieved.[2] However, in certain anatomical areas like the skull base,

Anshul Sama FRCS (for correspondence)
Consultant in Otorhinolaryngology, Department of Otorhinolaryngology, Head and Neck Surgery, Queen's Medical Centre, Nottingham University Hospital, Nottingham NG3 5DS, UK
E-mail: anshul.sama@nuh.nhs.uk

Nick S. Jones MD FRCS
Consultant in Otorhinolaryngology, Department of Otorhinolaryngology, Head and Neck Surgery, Queen's Medical Centre, Nottingham University Hospital, Nottingham NG3 5DS, UK
E-mail: nick.jones@nottingham.ac.uk

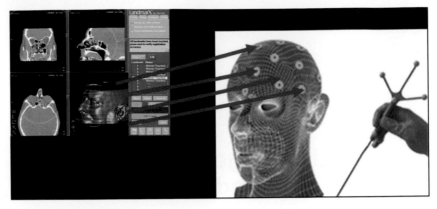

Fig. 1 Registration process.

pituitary fossa and the frontal recess, this degree of accuracy can rarely be achieved in practice. One reason is that however accurate a system is in practice (target registration error or TRG) differs from what is often quoted (fiducial localisation error and fiducial registration error).

Central to all image-guided systems is the process of acquiring pre-operative radiological data (CT or MRI) and matching this to the patient on the operative table. This is achieved by associating the pre-operative scan with certain markers (fiducials) and matching them on the peri-operative anatomy (registration; Fig. 1). In recent years, the most significant technological advancements have been in simplifying the registration process (*e.g.* contour-based registration; Fig 2) and making it more user-friendly (*e.g.* mask-based contour registration; Fig 3). Although the skin surface contours registration system has no 'fixed' markers (*i.e.* fiducials), it uses the surface contour matching to achieve the same principle. This alleviates the need for patients to have fiducial markers on them during the process of acquiring the radiological images.

However, although these developments improve the surgeon–computer workstation interface, what impact do they have on the main purpose of the

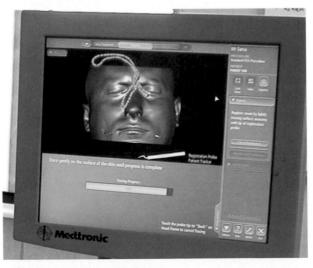

Fig. 2 Contour-based registration – Medtronic.

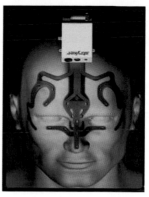

Fig. 3 Mask-based contour registration – Stryker.

IGS (*i.e.* accuracy). Target registration error (TRE) means the real difference between the position which the surgeon is in, compared to the image showing on the screen from the image-guidance system. This is the real and clinically important difference. Fiducial localisation error (FLE) is the mathematical error that occurs in the process of localising each individual marker or the contour of the patient in the operative situation. This occurs because of the errors associated with the tracking system, the difference in the pre- and peri-operative positions of the markers caused by soft tissue or head-set distortion and the human error involved in the placement of the probe on the fiducial markers. Post localisation of the individual markers registration is the process of 'best matching', the presumed location of the markers on the patient in the operative room with the location of the markers on the pre-operative scan. The best fit is achieved by mathematically calculating the alignment that minimises the differences between the pre- and peri-operative position of the markers. The fiducial registration error (FRE) is a representation of this mathematical factor used to achieve the best fit between the alignment readings during registration and the pre-operative radiological data (remember these data are not perfect in themselves). Most systems display the FRE post registration and most surgeons presume that this reflects the real-time accuracy (*i.e.* TRE of the system). Furthermore, achieving a lower FRE on the same or different patient using the same system does not translate into better accuracy. However, if the average FRE for many patients is lower for one system than another, using the same number of markers, it is likely that the system achieving the lower FRE is more accurate.

So how accurate are the current IGS systems? Most manufacturers and many published studies do not quote TRE figures because they are so variable. Whilst many studies may show that the majority of FRE readings have a mean accuracy of 1.5 mm,[3] it is important to realise that this is the mean value in a statistical distribution (χ^2 with three degrees of freedom). That is to say that 95% of the time the FRE will be 2.6 mm or better, and in 5% worse.[4] Reviewing the data on TRE gleamed from the most relevant articles in this area, it is clear that there is a lack of standardisation in reporting of accuracy and a discernible worsening in the TRE with laser skin contour and propriety head sets.

The problem with registration is in trying to match up the CT data (which may only be accurate to within 1–2 mm or more depending how the data are gathered), and the patient. Any registration that involves soft tissue registration or the use of a propriety head set is likely to have some distortion and inaccuracy between the pre- and peri-operative status. There are certain principles that reduce the error introduced. The more the number of markers/fiducials used, the better the accuracy of the system. The fiducials need to be widely dispersed, avoid collinear placement, be in different planes and surround the whole area of interest. Therefore, fiducials on the anterior surface of the face may give FRE readings that might make the surgeon believe that there is a mean degree of accuracy to within 2 mm; however, in a more distant plane such as posteriorly at the sphenoid and basi-occiput, away from the site of the fiducials, this degree of accuracy is likely to be much less.

There are other practical peri-operative factors that may compound the accuracy of these systems that include those with a head gear or head set becoming more inaccurate as these can slip, or that electromagnetic system data are distorted by some iron alloy or ferromagnetic object. In infra-red systems, the beam may be cut off by a physical interruption and the accuracy can also be affected by the position of the tracking system.

Technology is progressing but it is vital that the surgeon recognises the limitations of image-guided systems and accurately interpret the accuracy data provided. The degree of accuracy to date suggests that image-guided systems are a valuable tool for the rhinologist in endonasal endoscopic sinus surgery to confirm their anatomical position, but they are not yet accurate enough to operate by, or completely rely on. Although the current commercially available image-guided surgery systems do not account for peri-operative changes in tissue, the role of real-time MRI in the operating theatre with non-ferromagnetic instruments is being investigated, as is real-time CT. This would have particular potential where there is brain shift caused by tumour resection in skull base surgery, as it would account for changes that result during surgery. This is important, as it emphasises the need to use the current systems to help confirm the surgeon's anatomical position, and no more.

CT–MRI FUSION

Traditionally, navigation systems allow the surgeon to navigate using CT or MRI data sets. The technique of superimposing one type of data set onto another to create a composite image is called CT–MRI fusion. This technology is advantageous in areas such as the endoscopic management of skull base lesions. The technology allows surgeons to use the CT data to define the bony landmarks and the MRI data to get better soft tissue definition.

Advances in this technique not only allow simple fusion of the data sets but also control of the proportion of the superimposed data set. For instance, whilst operating in the sinuses or on the bony skull base, the displayed image can be set to be predominantly based on CT (Fig. 4) and gain the bony definition. Alternatively, it could be altered to predominantly MRI when operating within the cranium or tumour (Fig. 5). Furthermore, fusion technology is not limited to CT and MRI data bases only. It is feasible to integrate CT or MRI angiography and, in theory, positron emission tomography (PET) or functional MRI data as well. Therefore, it should be feasible to fuse more than two databases at the same time to develop integrated anatomical, vascular and functional images.

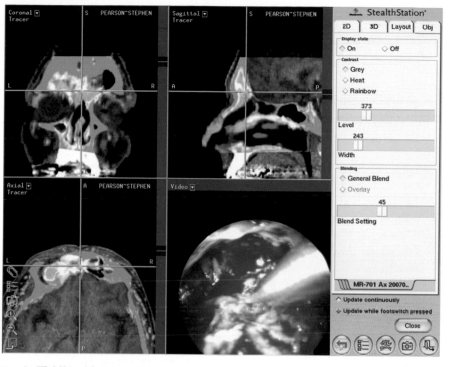

Fig. 4 CT–MRI with CT predominance in trans-sphenoidal pituitary surgery.

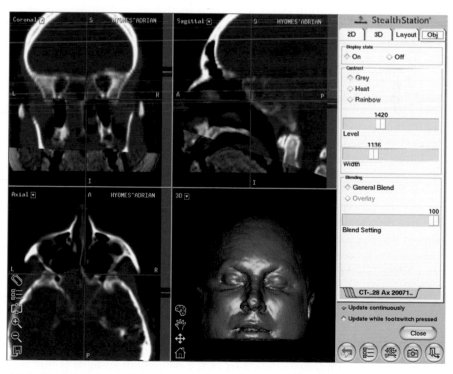

Fig. 5 CT–MRI fusion with MRI predominance in trans-sphenoidal pituitary surgery.

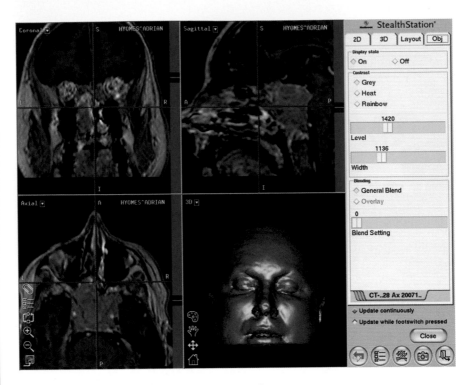

Fig. 6 CT–MRI fusion in pituitary giant macro-adenomas.

Fusion technology ideally lends itself to trans-sphenoidal pituitary surgery (Fig. 6). Access to the pituitary fossa through the sphenoid sinus needs the bony definition of CT images whilst the resection of the tumour would benefit from the better soft tissue definition of MRI. Having both data bases presented as a composite image would allow superior visualisation and overcome the limitations inherent in CT imaging alone. Integration of angiographic data is extremely useful when operating on large macro-adenomas with lateral extension, juvenile angiogfibromas, clivus cordomas and extended skull base approaches going lateral to carotid vessels.

Although such technological developments are extremely exciting, one should not loose sight of the limitations of the technology. The process of fusion is achieved by the same mathematical process as 'registration'. Registration involves the process of finding the best mathematical match between the pre-operative imaging data set (MRI or CT) and the patient on the operating table. Inherent in this process is an error, *i.e.* 'registration error'. Fusion uses a similar mathematical process to match the two data sets. Inherent in this is a further error factor. These fused data sets are then registered with the patient. There is no data available on the 'registration error' of fusing two data sets and the error in using fused data set for on-table registration.

INTRA-OPERATIVE UPDATING OF RADIOLOGICAL INFORMATION

One of the most significant limitations of the navigation systems is that it is reliant on pre-operative radiological data and is currently unable to reflect the intra-operative changes. As the systems will remain accurate for only those structures that remain in the same position as per the time of the registration, if the operation alters, removes or displaces the anatomical structures, the technology is unable to identify the change and the navigation effectively becomes outdated or inaccurate. This has been a major drawback in its use in neurosurgery for the phenomenon often called 'soft tissue shift'.

This drawback can be addressed by updating the pre-operative data with intra-operative imaging, *i.e.* fluoroscopy, CT or MRI. However, intra-operative imaging is not readily available and attempts at developing this technology have been limited by the cost implications and cumbersome nature of the apparatus. Although Fried *et al.*[5] found that real-time MRI may have some utility in sinus surgery, particularly when soft-tissue detail is essential, its current usage is limited to selected neurosurgical procedures, including trans-sphenoidal pituitary surgery. The development of smaller, more powerful magnets and greater automation within the operating room may make this technology more feasible in the future.

Few centres have attempted intra-operative CT, but the drawbacks are considerable because of concerns about radiation exposure and poor image quality.[6] Although fluoroscopy has the advantage of being cheaper with lower radiation, it is two-dimensional and has poorer image quality.[7]

TRACKING SYSTEMS

Early IGS systems used simple pointers with a fixed intra-operative localising device (ILD; array of LEDs or electromagnetic sensors) for intra-operative monitoring. These were replaced by ILDs that could be attached to a range of surgical instruments (*e.g.* suckers, drills, forceps, *etc.*). However, one of the limitations of IGS has been that it can only track a 'surgical device' with a fixed, rigid configuration. Traditionally, the surgical instrument would have a proximal ILD, *i.e.* the ILD is usually attached to the proximal end of the instrument in use. Although the specific instrument in use has been registered for the computer workstation to localise its tip correctly, any distortion of the instrument will result in a notable additional error and an increase in the TRE. Such distortions can become notable when working with curved instrumentation in confined bony spaces, such as a curved sucker in the frontal sinus (Fig. 7). Furthermore, IGS cannot be used with instruments that change configuration or are flexible.

An interesting development has been the introduction of distal ILDs as developed by the newly introduced Medtronic electromagnetic system (Fig. 8). This technology is only feasible with electromagnetic systems, as the ILD has to maintain visual continuity with the receiver for it to function in an optical system. This development opens up a new dimension of applications traditionally not available to IGS. Such technology will allow tracking of a flexible device in a human cavity or lumen. Possible applications can be tracking of endoscopes in body cavities, of catheters within the vascular tree and flexible endoscopes within the cranial ventricular system. In the realm of sinus surgery, it could increase the accuracy of the tracking by shortening the distance between the ILD and the operative site. However, this technology is still in its infancy and we await its development and the new applications it may present.

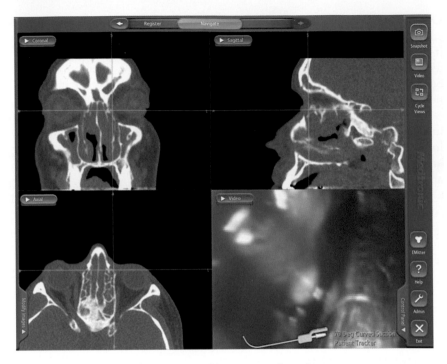

Fig. 7 Inaccurate tracking due to surgical instrument distortion.

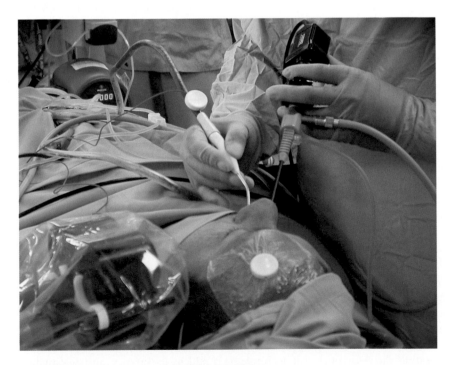

Fig. 8 Medtronic electromagnetic distal ILD probe.

CONCLUSIONS

Image-guidance systems should be seen as a way of improving intra-operative localisation of surgical instruments and should make the surgical procedure safer. It provides a better perception in three dimensions by way of its three planner scan display; in particular, it gives an increase in the perception of depth that is often lost with the use of the endoscope. It allows monitoring the proximity of essential landmarks to the position of instruments and re-inforces the surgeons' perception of their position in the operative field. However, although the data suggest accuracy within 2 mm, there is a need for caution on the degree of reliance attached to this figure and its use in situations where submillimetric precision is required. It is also essential that the surgeon understands the mathematical process of the registration and the inherent errors associated with this process. Today, IGS is used routinely for the most complex cases treated by ESS and for minimally invasive endoscopic approaches to the skull base. Clinical experiences suggest that, although CAS is not required for every case, it does offer significant advantages for the most complex cases (*e.g.* revision surgery, frontal and sphenoid sinus surgery, profuse polypopsis, tumours and skull base surgery). Nonetheless, IGS is not a substitute for thorough surgical training, knowledge of surgical anatomy, and sound intra-operative surgical decision making. Improvements in technology may lead to further improvements in accuracy, reliability, and utility and with this IGS may emerge as an indispensable component for advanced rhinological surgical techniques.

Key points for clinical practice

- Image-guided systems are a valuable tool to confirm anatomical position; however, they are not yet accurate enough to operate by, or completely rely on.

- CT–MRI fusion allows the definition of bony landmarks while enhancing soft tissue definition.

- Fusion technology which might include angiographic data would lend itself particularly well to trans-sphenoidal pituitary and extended skull base surgery.

- Development of real-time imaging systems could be invaluable with intra-operative anatomical changes and soft tissue shift.

- Although it is envisaged CAS would not be required in every case, it does offer significant advantages in the complex case.

References

1. International Society for Computer-Aided Surgery. *Computer-aided surgery: aims and scope.* Available at <www.iscas.net/>.
2. Roth M, Lanza DC, Zinreich J *et al.* Advantages and disadvantages of three-dimensional computed tomography intraoperative localization for functional endoscopic sinus surgery. *Laryngoscope* 1995; **105**: 1279–1286.

3. Schmerber S, Chassat F. Accuracy evaluation of a CAS system: laboratory protocol and results with 6D localizers, and clinical experiences in otorhinolaryngology. *Comput Aided Surg* 2001; **6**: 1–13.

4. Labadie RF, Davis BM, Fitzpatrick JM. Image guided surgery: what is the accuracy?. *Curr Opin Otolaryngol Head Neck Surg* 2005; **13**: 27–31.

5. Fried MP, Topulus G, Hsu L *et al*. Endoscopic sinus surgery with magnetic resonance imaging guidance: initial patient experience. *Otolaryngol Head Neck Surg* 1998; **119**: 374–380.

6. Cartellieri M, Vorbeck F. Endoscopic sinus surgery using intraoperative CT imaging for updating a three dimensional navigation system. *Laryngoscope* 2000; **110**: 292–296.

7. Brown SM, Sadougili BCH, Fried MP. Feasibility of real-time image-guided sinus surgery using intraoperative fluoroscopy. Presented at the American Rhinologic Society 2005 Annual Meeting. Los Angeles, CA: 24 September 2005.

Anu Daudia Nick S. Jones

11

Questioning the prevalence of chronic rhinosinusitis

When reviewing the current literature on chronic rhinosinusitis (CRS), it becomes clear that giving an accurate estimate of the prevalence of CRS is not straight-forward. This is, in part, because of the diversity of the disorders that encompass this category as well as the varied and imprecise diagnostic criteria that are sometimes used. CRS is estimated to be one of the most prevalent chronic diseases in the US, reportedly affecting 31 million patients each year.[1]

Data from the National Health Interview survey cite that it affects 14–16% in the US population based on a large probability sample survey conducted by trained interviewers.[2–5] The patients were asked to recall if they had ever been told by a physician or healthcare provider that they had chronic sinusitis defined as having 'sinus trouble' for more than 3 months in the year before the interview. In Canada, the prevalence of CRS, defined as an affirmative answer to the question 'Has the patient had sinusitis diagnosed by a health professional lasting for more than 6 months?' ranged from 3.4% in males to 5.7% in female subjects.[6] This method of estimating prevalence based on patient interviews is likely to overestimate the prevalence as it depends on the way the question is asked, relies on patient recall and whether an accurate diagnosis was made in the first place.

When looking at the diagnosis validated by a physician using ICD-9 codes as an identifier,[7] high prevalence has not been found and the figure was approximately 2%. This method of estimating prevalence relies on accurate diagnosis and may be limited by the physicians' speciality, level of training and the availability of equipment such as a rigid endoscope. The majority of

Anu Daudia FRCS
Specialist Registrar in Otolaryngology, Department of Otolaryngology, Head and Neck Surgery, Queen's Medical Centre, University of Nottingham, Nottingham NG7 2UH, UK

Nick S. Jones MD FRCS (for correspondence)
Professor of Otolaryngology, Department of Otolaryngology, Head and Neck Surgery, Queen's Medical Centre, University of Nottingham, Nottingham NG7 2UH, UK
E-mail: nick.jones@nottingham.ac.uk

primary care physicians do not have the training or equipment to perform nasal endoscopy which may lead to overdiagnosis.[8]

PROBLEMS WITH ARRIVING AT A DIAGNOSIS

In order to calculate the prevalence of chronic rhinosinusitis, an accurate diagnosis needs to be established. No consensus exists as to the optimal diagnostic algorithm for patients with CRS. In 1997, the American Academy of Otolaryngology–Head and Neck Surgery (AAO-HNS) convened the Rhinosinusitis Task Force to initiate a more rigorous analysis of the definition of CRS.[9] With regard to duration, 'chronic' rhinosinusitis was defined as having been present for a minimum of 12 weeks. In addition, the major and minor factors (symptoms and signs) associated with the diagnosis of CRS were elaborated. Major factors included facial pain/pressure, facial congestion/fullness, nasal obstruction/blockage, nasal discharge/coloured postnasal discharge, dysosmia, and purulence in the nasal cavity on examination. Minor factors were indicated including headache, fever (all non-acute), halitosis, fatigue, dental pain, cough, and ear pain/pressure/fullness. For the diagnosis of CRS, the task force indicated that two major factors or one major factor and two minor factors or purulence on examination constituted a strong history for CRS. However, they also stipulated that facial pain/pressure alone does not constitute a suggestive history for rhinosinusitis in the absence of other symptoms.

Subsequently, further task force initiatives have codified diagnostic criteria for CRS as well as serially summarising the evolving literature on the diagnosis and pathophysiology of CRS.[10,11] Despite such efforts, considerable controversies continue to evolve with respect to CRS.

As the diagnosis of CRS has primarily been based on symptoms, often excluding dysosmia, this often means that the diagnosis of CRS is often overestimated.[12] Recent studies have drawn attention to the problems in arriving at an accurate diagnosis of chronic rhinosinusitis.[13] Pynnonen and Terrel[13] found that 40% of those labelled as having chronic rhinosinusitis did not have the condition. These authors point out that all too often acute bacterial rhinosinusitis is confused with the more common viral upper respiratory tract infection and that a positive culture should be the gold standard for establishing the diagnosis. They emphasise the definition of CRS made by Lanza and Kennedy,[9] that there should be confirmation by nasal endoscopy,[14] computed tomography (CT) scans,[12] or both. Making a diagnosis of CRS without endoscopic or marked CT changes to support a clinical diagnosis on the basis of symptoms alone is unreliable. Interpretation of the appearance of sinuses on CT scans alone must be treated with caution as about 30% of asymptomatic patients will demonstrate mucosal thickening in one or more sinuses.[15,16] Furthermore, the extent of mucosal changes on CT has been shown not to correlate with the extent of patients' symptoms.[17]

There is increasing concern that CRS is overdiagnosed in patients with facial pain or pressure as when this is an isolated symptom, it is rarely caused by CRS.[18–21] Patients with facial pain or headache without nasal symptoms are very unlikely to be helped by nasal medical or surgical treatment.[20,22] Patients with facial pain often make a self-diagnosis of 'sinusitis', because they know

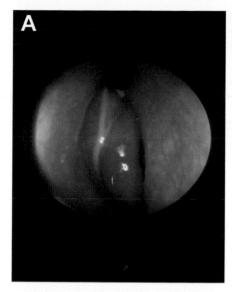
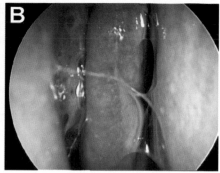

Fig. 1 (A) Endoscopic changes of chronic infective rhinosinusitis. (B) Chronic rhinosinusitis without infection.

that their sinuses lie within the face. In the medical literature, rhinological causes of facial pain include acute infective rhinosinusitis – typically preceded by an upper respiratory tract infection, which is often short-lived. Chronic infective rhinosinusitis has been assumed to be the most common cause of most patients' chronic facial pain but, with the advent of nasal endoscopy and computerised tomography, along with the finding that in many patients facial pain persists after endoscopic sinus surgery,[20,23,24] it has become apparent that this is not the case. It is notable that more than 80% of patients with purulent secretions visible at nasal endoscopy have no facial pain.[20] Many patients who report intermittent symptoms of facial pain, which they think is due to infection, are found to have no evidence of infection on nasal endoscopy when symptomatic in clinic. Often, a neurological cause for their facial pain is responsible. In cases of facial pain secondary to genuine sinusitis, it is rare not to have endoscopic signs of disease (Fig. 1A,B).[14] Patients with CRS almost invariably have co-existing symptoms of nasal obstruction, hyposmia, and/or a purulent nasal discharge.[25] In this group of patients with genuine sinusitis, endoscopic sinus surgery has been shown to alleviate facial pain in 75–83% of cases.[20,26] Other causes of facial pain include atypical forms of migraine,[27] cluster headache, paroxysmal hemicrania,[28] atypical facial pain,[29,30] and midfacial segment pain.[22]

MIDFACIAL SEGMENT PAIN

Midfacial segment pain has all the characteristics of tension-type headache, except that it affects the midface. Patients describe a feeling of pressure, heaviness or tightness and they may say that their nose feels blocked when they have no airway obstruction. The symptoms are symmetrical and may involve the nasion, the bridge of the nose, either side of the nose, the peri-orbital region, retro-orbitally or across the cheeks. The forehead and occipital region may also be affected at the same time in about 60% of patients. There are no consistent exacerbating or relieving factors and patients often take a range of analgesics, which have no, or a minimal, effect other than Ibuprofen that may help a few to a minor extent. The symptoms are often initially episodic but are often persistent by the time they are seen in secondary care. Patients may be convinced that their symptoms are due to sinusitis as they know that their sinuses lie under this area with the exception of the bridge of the nose. They may have been treated for a long period with antibiotics and topical nasal steroids and a few patients have had some transient response on occasions that may be related to the placebo effect or cognitive dissonance, but these are inconsistent. Patients' symptoms are not worse with routine physical activity, and rarely interfere with the patient getting to sleep.

To make matters more complex, the stimulus of a genuine acute sinus infection may exacerbate the symptoms, with a return to the background face ache on resolution of the infection. It is hardly surprising that patients (and doctors) will interpret all their symptoms as being related to their sinuses. Patients often describe tenderness on touching the areas of the forehead or cheeks leading them to think there is underlying inflammation of the bone. However, on examination, there is hyperesthesia of the skin and soft tissues in these areas and gently touching these is enough to cause discomfort and there is no evidence of underling bony disease. This is similar to the tender areas over the forehead and scalp seen with tension-type headache. It appears that this is an organic disorder as an increase in the pain sensitivity in the central nervous system has been found in tension-type headache.[31] Nasal endoscopy is normal. As approximately 1 in 3 asymptomatic people have incidental changes on CT scan, this may confuse the picture. A trial of maximal nasal medical treatment including oral and nasal steroids and a broad-spectrum antibiotic with anaerobic cover fails to help their symptoms. The majority of patients with this condition respond to low-dose amitriptyline after a period of 6 weeks.

If amitriptyline fails, then relief may be obtained from gabapentin, pregabalin, propranolol, carbamazepine and, occasionally, sodium valproate. It seems likely that the underlying pathology in midfacial segment pain is similar to tension-type headache. The aetiology of this type of pain is uncertain but Olesen's theory[32,33] that integrates the effects of myofascial afferents, the activation of peripheral nociceptors and their convergence on the caudal nucleus of trigeminal, along with qualitative changes in the central nervous system, provides one of the best models. There is also a suggestion that there is a down-regulation of central inhibition from supraspinal impulses due to psychological stress and emotional disturbances. Other mechanisms have been proposed that include sensitisation of peripheral myofascial receptors, sensitisation of second-order neurons at the spinal or trigeminal level, sensitisation of supraspinal neurons or decreased antinociceptive activity from supraspinal structures.[34] The trigeminal caudal nucleus is the major relay nucleus for head and neck pain, and it appears that supraspinal excitatory input contributes to intense neuronal activation resulting in a generalised increase in sensitivity of the nociceptive pathways, both centrally and peripherally. Midfacial segment pain may be a state of trigeminal neuronal hypersensitivity and pain facilitation. Olesen's model is attractive as it might explain much of the clinical picture of midfacial segment pain;[32] for example, the skin and soft-tissue hyperaesthesia that accompanies the pain may be due to the above hypersensitivity of the pain pathways. It is of interest that, if surgery is mistakenly performed as a treatment for midfacial segment pain, the pain may sometimes abate temporarily, only to return after several weeks to months.

CONCLUSIONS

The prevalence of chronic rhinosinusitis is widely quoted to be around 14–16% in the US population. However, giving an accurate estimate of the prevalence of CRS is not straight-forward because of the diversity of the disorders that encompass this category as well as the varied and imprecise diagnostic criteria that are sometimes used. Another confounding factor is that the diagnostic criteria include symptoms with endoscopy or CT changes and, given the high prevalence of incidental changes on CT in an asymptomatic population, this too will lead to overdiagnosis. Making a diagnosis of CRS without endoscopic signs or marked CT changes to support a clinical diagnosis on the basis of symptoms alone is unreliable as is a diagnosis that is based on minor CT changes alone. When looking at a diagnosis validated by a physician using ICD-9 codes as an identifier, the prevalence was found to be approximately 2%. If facial pain and pressure are the primary symptoms in the absence of any nasal symptoms or signs (normal nasal endoscopy), it is unlikely to be due to sinus disease. These patients may have an incorrect diagnosis of chronic rhinosinusitis and may well have neuralgic types of facial pain such as midfacial segment pain.

Key points for clinical practice

- Providing an accurate estimate of the prevalence of chronic rhinosinusitis is not straight-forward because of the diversity of the disorders that encompass the symptoms that are associated with this condition as well as the varied and imprecise diagnostic criteria that are sometimes used.

- If facial pain and pressure are the primary symptoms, sinus disease in the absence of any nasal symptoms or signs is unlikely. These patients can be incorrectly labelled as having chronic rhinosinusitis and are more likely to have neuralgic types of facial pain such as midfacial segment pain.

- Patients with facial pain in addition to nasal obstruction, a loss of sense of smell, and the following symptoms – worse with a cold, flying, or skiing – might be helped by nasal medical or surgical treatment.

- The majority of patients seen in a rhinological clinic with pain are found to be due to causes other than sinusitis.

(continued)

Key points for clinical practice *(continued)*

- Patients with normal nasal endoscopy are unlikely to have pain due to rhinosinusitis.

- Patients with a normal CT scan are unlikely to have pain due to rhinosinusitis (note that approximately 33% of asymptomatic patients have incidental mucosal changes on CT and, therefore, radiographic changes alone are not diagnostic of symptomatic rhinosinusitis).

References

1. Meltzer EO, Hamilos DL, Hadley JA *et al*. Rhinosinusitis: establishing definitions for clinical research and patient care. *J Allergy Clin Immunol* 2006; **118 (Suppl)**: S17–S61.
2. Benson V, Marano MA. *Current Estimates From The National Health Interview Survey, 1995 Vital and Health Statistics*. Hyattsville, MD: National Centre for Health Statistics, 1995; 199: 1–428.
3. Collins JG. *Prevalence of selected chronic conditions: United States, 1990–1992*. Hyattsville, MD: National Centre for Health Statistics, 1997; 194: 1–89.
4. Blackwell DCJ, Coles R. *Summary health statistics for US adults: National Health Interview Survey 1997*. Hyattsville, MD: National Centre for Health Statistics, 2002; 205: 15.
5. Cherry DK, Woodwell DA. *National Ambulatory Care Survey: 2000 Summary*. Hyattsville, MD: National Centre for Health Statistics 2000; 328: 1–32.
6. Chen Y, Dales R, Lin M. The epidemiology of chronic rhinosinusitis in Canadians. *Laryngoscope* 2003; **113**: 1199–1205.
7. Shashy RG, Moore EJ, Weaver A. Prevalence of chronic sinusitis diagnosis in Olmsted County, Minnesota. *Arch Otolaryngol Head Neck Surg* 2004; **130**: 320–323.
8. Bonfils P, Halimi P, Bihan CL, Nores J-M, Avan P, Landais P. Correlation between nasosinusal symptoms and tomographic diagnosis in chronic rhinosinusitis. *Ann Otol Laryngol* 2005; **114**: 74–83.
9. Lanza D, Kennedy DW. Adult rhinosinusitis defined. *Otolaryngol Head Neck Surg* 1997; **117 (Suppl)**: S1–S7.
10. Benninger MS. Adult chronic rhinosinusitis: definitions, diagnosis, epidemiology, and pathophysiology. *Otolaryngol Head Neck Surg* 2003; **129 (Suppl)**: S1–S32.
11. Meltzer EO, Hamilos DL, Hadley JA **et al**. Rhinosinusitis: establishing definitions for clinical research and patient care. *Otolaryngol Head Neck Surg* 2004; **131 (Suppl)**: S1–S62.
12. Bhattacharyya N. Clinical and symptom criteria for the accurate diagnosis of chronic rhinosinusitis. *Laryngoscope* 2006; **116 (Suppl 110)**: 1–22.
13. Pynnonen MA, Terrell JE. Conditions that masquerade as chronic rhinosinusitis: a medical record review. *Otolaryngol Head Neck Surg* 2006; **132**: 748–751.
14. Hughes R, Jones NS. The role of endoscopy in outpatient management. *Clin Otolaryngol* 1998; **23**: 224–226.
15. Marshall A, Jones NS. The utility of radiological studies in the diagnosis and management of rhinosinusitis. *Curr Infect Dis Report* 2003; **5**: 199–204.
16. Jones NS. A review of the CT staging systems, the prevalence of anatomic variations, incidence of mucosal findings and their correlation with symptoms, surgical and pathological findings. *Clin Otolaryngol* 2002; **27**: 171–174.
17. Bhattacharya T, Piccirillo J, Wippold FJ. Relationship between patient-based descriptions of sinusitis and paranasal sinus computed tomographic findings. *Arch Otolaryngol Head Neck Surg* 1997; **123**: 1189–1192.
18. Stewart MG. Sinus pain: is it real? *Curr Opin Otolaryngol Head Neck Surg* 2002; **10**: 29–32.
19. Paulson EP, Graham SM. Neurologic diagnosis and treatment in patients with computed tomography and nasal endoscopy negative facial pain. *Laryngoscope* 2004; **11**: 992–996.

20. West B, Jones NS. Endoscopy-negative, computed tomography-negative facial pain in a nasal clinic. *Laryngoscope* 2001; **111**: 581–586.
21. Jones NS. Midfacial segment pain: implications for rhinitis and rhinosinusitis. *Curr Allergy Asthma Report* 2004; **4**: 187–192.
22. Hessler JL, Piccirillo JF, Fang D *et al.* Clinical outcomes of chronic rhinosinusitis in response to medical therapy: results of a prospective study. *Am J Rhinol* 2007; **21**: 10–18.
23. Tarabichi M. Characteristics of sinus-related pain. *Otolaryngol Head Neck Surg* 2000; **122**: 84–87.
24. Jones NS, Cooney TR. Facial pain and sinonasal surgery. *Rhinology* 2003; **41**: 193–200.
25. Fahy C, Jones NS. Nasal polyposis and facial pain. *Clin Otolaryngol* 2001; **26**: 510–513.
26. Acquadro MA, Salan SD, Joseph MP. Analysis of pain and endoscopic sinus surgery for sinusitis. *Ann Otol Rhinol Laryngol* 1997; **106**: 305–309.
27. Daudia AT, Jones NS. Facial migraine in a rhinological setting. *Clin Otolaryngol* 2002; **27**: 251–255.
28. Fuad F, Jones NS. Is there an overlap between paroxysmal hemicrania and cluster headache? *J Laryngol Otol* 2002; **27**: 472–479.
29. Jones NS. Facial pain and headache. In: Kerr A, Mackay IS, Bull TR. (eds) *Scott Brown's Otolaryngology*, vol 4, 6th edn. London: Butterworths, 1996; 1–10.
30. Jones NS. The classification and diagnosis of facial pain. *Hosp Med* 2001; **62**: 598–606.
31. Ashina A, Bendtsen L, Ashina M, Magrel W, Jensen R. Generalised hyperalgesia in patients with chronic tension-type headache. *Cephalgia* 2006; **26**: 940–948.
32. Olesen J. Clinical and pathophysiological observations in migraine and tension type headache explained by integration of vascular, supraspinal and myofascial inputs. *Pain* 1991; **46**: 125–132.
33. Jensen R, Olesen J. Tension-type headache: an update on mechanisms and treatment. *Curr Opin Neurol* 2000; **13**: 285–289.
34. Bendtsen L, Jensen R, Olesen J. Quantitatively altered nociception in chronic myofascial pain. *Pain* 1996; **65**: 259–264.

James Keir Ray Clarke

12

New treatments in recurrent respiratory papillomatosis

Recurrent respiratory papillomatosis (RRP) is a chronic relapsing condition characterised by multiple warty exophytic lesions on the mucosal surface of the respiratory tract (Fig. 1). RRP is now known to be caused by the human papilloma virus (HPV). An intranuclear virus is evident in lesions by electron microscopy and HPV DNA may be found in laryngeal papillomas using southern blot hybridisation.[1] Viral probes have identified HPV in virtually every papilloma lesion studied.[2] The virus is a small, DNA containing, capsid virus with a double-stranded, supercoiled, circular DNA.

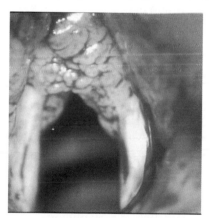

Fig. 1 Typical appearance of RRP in the larynx (courtesy of Dr Andrew Bowhay, Consultant Anaesthetist, Royal Liverpool Children's Hospital, Alder Hey).

James Keir MRCS DOHNS (for correspondence)
Specialist Registrar in Otolaryngology, Royal Liverpool Children's Hospital, Alder Hey, Liverpool, UK
E-mail: jameskeir@hotmail.com

Ray Clarke BSc DCH FRCS FRCS(ORL)
Consultant in Otolaryngology, Royal Liverpool Children's Hospital, Alder Hey, Liverpool, UK

The HPV is separated into types based on the viral genome.[2] HPV type 6 and type 11 are the most common aetiological agents. Type 11 conveys a particularly aggressive course to RRP which can result in conversion to squamous cell carcinoma.[3] The disease occurs in adults and in children, where it is known as juvenile onset recurrent respiratory papillomatosis (JORRP). Viral transmission in children is thought to occur primarily from the birth canal of HPV-infected mothers but host susceptibility plays an important part in aetiology. Both humoral and cellular responses may be compromised in children with RRP, which in turn may also influence the clinical course of the disease.[4]

Presentation is typically between the ages of 2–4 years but JORRP has been described in 1-day-old children.[5] Hoarseness is the predominant presenting symptom but children can present with stridor due to airway obstruction. Girls and boys are equally affected. The prevalence in the US and Danish populations has been calculated as 4.3 and 3.62 in 100,000 children, respectively.[5,6]

Lesions may occur anywhere in the respiratory tract, most commonly the larynx. Typically, the glottic epithelium at the squamocolumnar junction is involved. There is a large variation in disease severity. Some children develop single, slow-growing lesions that require infrequent endoscopic removal to improve voice. At the severe end of the disease spectrum, children develop rapidly progressive fatal airway obstruction. The most important prognostic indicator is the age at diagnosis with patients younger than 3 years of age requiring significantly more frequent surgery. Younger children are also more likely to have multicentric disease and to need tracheostomy.[7] Severely affected children show rapid proliferative disease with life-threatening encroachment on the airway and need frequent, in some cases weekly, removal of bulky disease to avoid tracheostomy. Unexplained remissions occur and the disease course can be unpredictable. Tracheobronchial spread is a rare but ominous development and subsequent progression to carcinoma of the bronchus is well documented.[8]

JORRP can have a major adverse influence on quality of life for children and families. This is due not only to the disabling symptoms but because children often require multiple hospital stays with a reported average of 4.4 surgical procedures per child per year.[9] Severely affected children are at risk of sudden deterioration and may require multiple unpredicted as well as scheduled admissions. JORRP is a potentially fatal disease. Management of even a small number of children with JORRP can be a significant burden on resources for a children's ENT service. Derkay[5] calculated the annual economic burden of treatment of RRP in the US in 1995 at $150 million.

The mainstay of current management is surgery with endoscopic removal of macroscopic disease, repeated as dictated by rapidity of progression in each case. The desired outcomes are preservation of voice and maintenance of the airway. Tracheostomy must be avoided if at all possible and most parents/carers and otolaryngologists will opt for multiple, frequent admissions for local disease control rather than tracheostomy. The morbidity and potential mortality of this procedure is well known but in JORRP there is the added concern that it may promote tracheobronchial disease spread.[10] This is thought to arise because tracheostomy creates a squamocolumnar junction

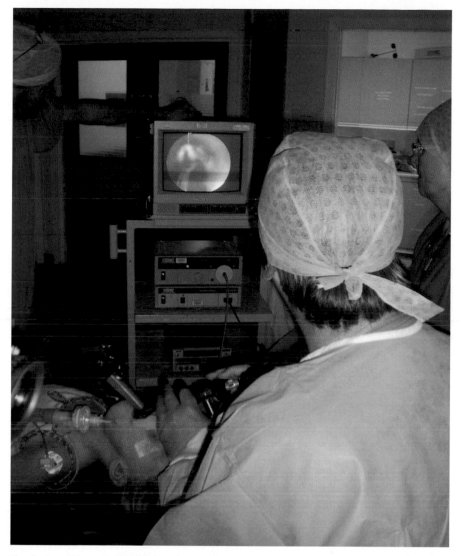

Fig. 2 A patient prepared for endoscopic surgery with surgeon assessing extent of disease with endoscope on screen.

that facilitates viral spread; however, children who require this intervention will inevitably have more aggressive disease.

A variety of adjuvant therapies may be used in an attempt to prolong the interval between endoscopic treatments, to reduce the risk of tracheobronchial spread and to ensure avoidance of tracheostomy. More recent work focuses on the potential for disease prevention by vaccination against the human papilloma virus.

SURGERY

Prior to the development of endoscopic laryngeal surgery and of paediatric anaesthetic and peri-operative care techniques that permit such surgery, RRP

157

in children was frequently fatal. Early surgical techniques included cold steel dissection of gross lesions, suction diathermy, cryosurgery and ultrasonography. Apart from cold steel dissection, these techniques have been largely superseded.

Modern endolaryngeal surgical instruments have made cold steel dissection much easier and safer, with a low risk of scar formation. For isolated lesions with a defined pedicle, this is still the technique of choice for many surgeons. Unlike 'hot' techniques, there is no virus-containing vapour plume but bleeding can obscure the surgeon's view and may facilitate seeding of viral particles.[1,2] Moreover, suitable lesions where there is a defined pedicle are uncommon and the more usual presentation of multiple, broad-based, warty lesions with frequent and rapid recurrence makes this approach impractical.

Hence the two mainstays of modern surgical management are laser ablation and the powered microdebrider.

LASER SURGERY

Laser surgery was a major advance in the management of RRP and was popularised for laryngeal surgery by Strong in the 1970s.[11] A laser works on the principle that energy is absorbed by water in tissues, leading to destruction and cauterisation of surface tissues with minimal thermal injury to adjacent areas. Most lasers are combined with an infrared or 'aiming' beam which enables the surgeon to direct the laser precisely. When coupled with an operating microscope, the laser gives a precise, controlled method of vapourising lesions.

Lasers are classified mainly by the type of gas used to generate the beam, for example, CO_2 and potassium-titanyl-phosphate (KTP). Because of its excellent haemostatic control and precision, the laser most commonly used in laryngeal surgery is the CO_2 laser. It is the standard laser for RRP management.[2,12] A significant disadvantage of the CO_2 laser is that the beam cannot be delivered through a flexible fibre endoscope. The KTP laser can be used in this way and, although it is more cumbersome and less precise, it is more suitable for distal tracheobronchial disease. A small number of surgeons also use pulsed dye laser, pump dye laser and argon plasma coagulation.[2,12]

There are important safety concerns with the laser. Inadvertent injury to normal tissue has been described. Despite its apparent precision, there may be damage to a small zone of tissue beyond the area of application and iatrogenic scarring and webbing, particularly in the anterior commisure, may occur.

Healthcare staff who use the laser or are in theatre during its use must have specific training. Precautions such as wet drapes, modifications to anaesthetic and endotracheal equipment and protective eye-wear for theatre personnel are mandatory.

When used with volatile anaesthetic agents and oxygen, there is a risk of airway combustion with resultant often-catastrophic damage to normal structures. As awareness of the potential for airway fires has increased, the training of theatre personnel has improved and protocols for safe laser surgery have developed, this is now an extremely rare event.[13]

Viral particles have been demonstrated in laser plume.[14] It has been hypothesised that these particles are potentially infective and could contribute to seeding or to infection of healthcare workers.[15]

MICRODEBRIDER

A rotary dissector was first used by Urban in acoustic neuroma surgery and in 1994 a powered instruments known as the 'hummer' was used in endonasal surgery. These combined a suction tip with an integrated rapidly rotating blade.[16] The combination of atraumatic dissection, minimal bleeding, and the ability to direct the tips of these instruments under endoscopic control made them especially suitable for endoscopic nasal surgery.[17] A further advantage was that the instrument selectively works on polypoid tissue and inadvertent damage to surrounding normal tissue is minimised (Fig. 3).

Powered instrumentation was first reported in the treatment of RRP at the turn of the century[18] with an angled-tip 3.5-mm blade facilitating its use in the larynx.[19] The microdebrider is used with the aid of a rigid, hand-held telescope with a video system and a monitor although some surgeons prefer the operating microscope. Reduced bleeding, better voice quality, less pain and reduced scarring have been reported. The microdebrider can be manoeuvred to reach subglottic and tracheal lesions and disease adjacent to an endotracheal tube, areas that are especially challenging for laser surgery.[19–21]

Powered instruments are relatively easy to learn to use. In contrast with the laser, the technique can be easily taught to surgeons in training without the

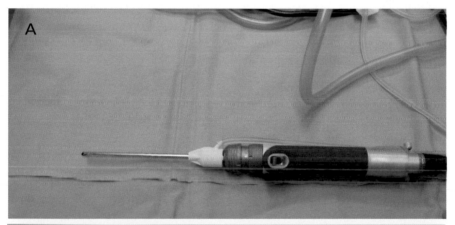

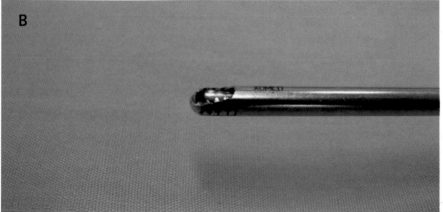

Fig. 3 (A,B) An example of a microdebrider with a close-up of the rotating blade.

need for external accreditation courses. Surgery tends to be quicker and better tolerated with a high degree of parental acceptance. The microdebrider is now the preferred surgical modality among otolaryngologists for the routine treatment of RRP in the US.[2] It was second only to the CO_2 laser in the UK up to 2004[12] but has now become the preferred first-line technique.

TRACHEOSTOMY

A very small proportion of children with JORRP will require tracheostomy, although this procedure is avoided if at all possible. It must be considered in children with rampant disease who do not respond to conventional measures including adjuvant treatments as detailed below and in whom airway obstruction is already established or imminent. Tracheostomy patients tend to have a worse prognosis, although it is noted that it is these children that often present at a younger age and with more widespread disease, *i.e.* the cohort of children who undergo tracheostomy have more aggressive disease.[10] There has been no change in tracheostomy rate in the US over two surveys carried out among members of the American Society of Pediatric Otolaryngology (ASPO) in 1994 and 2004.[22] The predilection of disease for squamocolumnar junctions means viral particles may colonise the tracheostomy site and lead to significant problems including distal spread. Decannulation should be considered as soon as management with endoscopic techniques is thought to be possible.

ANAESTHESIA AND PERI-OPERATIVE CARE

Paediatric anaesthesiology is now a discrete subspecialty that has contributed greatly to advances in the management of children with airway disorders. Peri-operative care of children has improved and day-case management of children with JORRP is increasingly the norm in specialised centres. Anaesthetic techniques vary and include spontaneous ventilation, apnoeic excision, endotracheal intubation and jet ventilation or combinations of the above.[5,12] A laser-safe endotracheal tube must be used when undertaking laser excision. In the apnoea technique, the child is intubated with an endotracheal tube and given 100% oxygen for a period. The child is then extubated and the surgeon is free to carry on further excision of papillomata without the inconvenience of having the tube in such a small airway. If necessary, the patient is re-intubated and re-oxygenated.

In jet ventilation, the anaesthetic gases are administered at high pressure through a tube usually clipped to the side of the surgeon's laryngoscope and at some distance to the laryngeal introitus. In this way, the glottis is not obscured by an endotracheal tube and the surgeon is free to work on the larynx. Surgery may be interrupted intermittently to permit 'jet' ventilation at high pressures. The technique is less commonly used nowadays. It may be implicated in distal spread of disease and there is a risk of pneumothorax.[23]

The authors' preference is to remove the bulk of disease with an endotracheal tube *in situ* and to complete the procedure with the child extubated and breathing spontaneously with the endotracheal tube in the pharynx. This involves close co-operation between surgeon and anaesthetist. Bleeding is reduced by placing 1 in 10,000 topical adrenaline on neurosurgical patties in the surgical field before and after application of the microdebrider. Optimum anaesthetic and peri-operative care requires a high degree of training and specialisation for both the surgeon and the anaesthetist.

Glucocorticoids have greatly improved the management of children with acute airway obstruction. This is presumably due to their anti-inflammatory effect in reducing laryngotracheal mucosal oedema.[24,25] This has led to consideration of the use of steroids when treating children with JORRP. The counter argument is that glucocorticoids are anti-inflammatory and, theoretically, may attenuate host defence mechanisms, thus promoting viral spread. There is no definite evidence to support this and many teams now give a single dose of peri-operative dexamethasone which seems to facilitate smooth recovery from anaesthesia. It is the authors' practice to recommend to parents of children with severe disease that they give the child a single dose (0.4 mg/kg body weight) of dexamethasone should the child develop any signs of airway obstruction (*e.g.* stridor or laboured breathing).

Photodocumentation of laryngeal pathology in children has improved greatly in recent years. A careful rigid endoscopic examination with pictorial recording of the findings is now standard. Parents will expect to be shown 'before' and 'after' views of the child's larynx. Although Derkay *et al.*[26] proposed a staging system for JORRP, many find it cumbersome to use and high-quality image capture is a more widely accepted way to monitor progress and response to treatment.

CENTRALISATION OF CARE

The low prevalence of JORRP limits the numbers of patients that are treated in any one institution. In a UK survey, the median number of children undergoing regular treatment per team was five, and in the US nine.[12,22] Sporadic treatment of very small numbers of children in departments that do not have dedicated paediatric anaesthetists and otolaryngologists with a special interest in this condition is difficult to justify. National registers of new cases have been proposed and would have the merit of allowing better documentation of response to new treatments.

ADJUVANT THERAPIES

RRP is a viral disease. Viral material is widely distributed in the respiratory epithelium of affected children and is found in macroscopically normal tissue.[27] While surgery is the mainstay of modern treatment, its role is inevitably limited to debulking disease and maintaining the child's airway and voice while waiting for disease remission. Currently, non-operative treatments are used as an adjunct to surgery but developments in basic science and in understanding of the precise aetiology of RRP may facilitate curative, non-surgical treatments. Currently, some 20% of children have some form of adjunctive treatment.[22]

The natural history of JORRP can be unpredictable, with periods of increased disease activity interspersed with good disease control and sometimes unexplained spontaneous remissions. This coupled with the rarity of the disease and the wide geographic distribution of cases has made evaluation of interventions very difficult, particularly the potentially toxic treatments that are only considered for children with severe disease. Hence, the evidence-base for most treatments is poor.

CONTROL OF GASTRO-OESOPHAGEAL REFLUX

Gastro-oesophageal reflux (GOR) is implicated in a variety of laryngeal pathologies in children and is thought to facilitate disease progression in JORRP. Injury to the respiratory mucosa in uncontrolled GOR may explain the observation that RRP is more aggressive in combination with this condition.[28] In children undergoing surgery, GOR has been purported to increase the number of soft tissue complications such as scarring and web formation. While the evidence for a long-term effect is uncertain, it seems prudent to screen children with JORRP for pathological reflux and treat it if it is present. Non-medical measures such as altering the sleeping position, antacids, H_2-receptor blockers and proton pump inhibitors have been used, with surgery (fundoplication) reserved for severe cases that fail to respond to less invasive interventions. High-dose cimetidine is thought to have an immunomodulatory side-effect independent of its anti-reflux effect. Unfortunately, the evidence-base for this remains uncertain.[29]

CIDOFOVIR

Cidofovir is a nucleoside analogue that acts against the herpes virus family and has been shown to induce apoptosis and augment immune responses.[30,31] Its mechanism of action is through the active intracellular metabolite cidofovir dehydrate which inhibits cytomegalovirus DNA polymerase. Cidofovir was developed for the systemic treatment of cytomegalovirus in HIV. Intralesional cidofovir was first given to an adult patient with squamous papilloma in the oesophagus–hypopharynx in 1995[32] and subsequently used in JORRP in 1999.[33] It has also been used systemically and in a nebulised form.[34] The response is often dramatic with, in some cases, complete resolution of advanced disease. Intralesional cidofovir has become the most widely used adjuvant therapy in children.

Several studies have shown an improvement in the interval time between surgical procedures. However, they involved small numbers of children and were not randomised, controlled or blinded.[35] Chetri *et al.*[36] treated five patients with intralesional injections of cidofovir at a concentration of 1 mg/ml at 2-weekly intervals for four treatments with the interval between treatments extended by 1 week after each subsequent treatment. After 9 weeks of treatment, no patients required further laser surgery. The mean papilloma stage decreased within 2 weeks of the first injection, and continued to decrease for the remainder of the 66-week follow-up period. Other studies have used cidofovir at the higher dose of 5 mg/ml with varying schedules of administration. The Pransky *et al.*[37] study in 2003 reported 11 patients who had all previously required surgical debulking at 2–6 week intervals demonstrating partial remission in five, complete remission in five and one patient who continued to require treatment.

In a more recently reported study with a mean follow-up of 30 months, 11 children were treated with intralesional cidofovir. Five required no further treatment, four had an initial remission but relapsed and two had no apparent response. The authors counsel caution concerning the potential long-term carcinogenic effects of cidofovir.[38]

Systemic cidofovir is toxic. Intralesional administration does not appear to produce systemic toxicity or local side-effects and plasma levels are below those leading to toxicity in children.[39] Caution has been raised in animal studies that have demonstrated the possibility of nephrotoxicity, carcinogenesis and hypospermia at doses currently used in humans, although thus far only a handful of cases in which cidofovir has been used have resulted in dysplasia and/or malignant transformation.[40] Histological findings in a small cohort of paediatric patients in which cidofovir had been administered did not demonstrate any dysplastic changes.[41] It is suggested that a frank discussion take place between physician and patient over the possible side-effects of the administration of cidofovir including the potential for carcinogenesis.[42]

INTERFERON

Interferon is the second most frequently used adjuvant therapy among otolaryngologists in the UK and US.[12,22] The interferons are a class of naturally occurring proteins produced by human leukocytes in response to a variety of stimuli including viral infection. They are manufactured commercially by recombinant DNA technology. They act by binding to specific membrane receptors and altering cell metabolism through antiviral, antiproliferative and immunomodulatory effects. The mechanisms are thought to be through blocking the viral replication of nucleic acids (RNA and DNA) and by altering cell membranes making them less susceptible to viral penetration. Interferons were discovered in 1957 by Isaacs and Lindenmann[43] and first used therapeutically in a Scandinavian trial in 1976. Haglund et al.[44] reported the first encouraging results with RRP in 1981.

Interferon-α may be administered subcutaneously or intravenously. In 1988, Healy et al.[45] reported a multicentre, randomised, controlled trial with 123 RRP patients randomised to receive treatment with surgery plus interferon or surgery alone. Interferon (2×10^6 IU/m^2 of body surface area) was given once daily for a week and then three times per week for 1 year. Treatment was followed up by a year of observation without the drug. Both study groups underwent serial endoscopy to remove papillomas and to document the efficacy of treatment. During the first 6 months, the growth rate of papillomas in the interferon group was significantly lower than in the control group ($P = 0.0007$). This difference was not sustained during the second 6 months and ceased to be statistically significant ($P = 0.68$). It was, therefore, suggested that interferon is neither a curative agent nor of substantial value as an adjunctive agent in the long term. Other multicentre studies,[46] however, have suggested that interferon had a significantly beneficial effect and that compared against historical controls, a statistically significant longer period of relapse-free survival is reported ($P = 0.001$).[47] It is noted that these multicentre studies give contradictory results and that the role of interferon in JORRP remains uncertain.

Interferon is associated with significant morbidity and potential mortality. The side-effects include acute toxicity with transient fever, fatigue, nausea, arthralgia and headache. Chronic reactions include elevation of serum transaminase levels, decreased growth rate of the child, leukopenia, spastic diplegia and febrile seizures. Interferon produced by recombinant DNA techniques has been reported as having fewer side-effects and better efficacy than blood-bank harvested interferon.[2]

RIBAVIRIN

Ribavirin is a broad-spectrum antiviral drug that is most commonly used to treat respiratory syncytial virus.[48] It is administered in an oral form or as an aerosol. Side-effects are common in the oral form and include headache, fatigue and anaemia. In its aerosol form, it achieves high local tissue concentrations without inducing side-effects. Its clinical efficacy in JORRP is uncertain. Studies have been non-randomised and with small numbers of patients.[49,50]

ACYCLOVIR

Acyclovir is nucleoside analogue. Its antiviral activity is dependent on the presence of virally encoded thymidine kinase. This is, however, an enzyme that is not encoded by papilloma virus so there is no plausible biological reason for a direct inhibitory effect in JORRP. It has been postulated that co-disease factors susceptible to the drug may be present. Viral co-infections with herpes simplex type 1, cytomegalovirus and Epstein–Barr virus have been detected in patients with RRP and progression of RRP in adults has been linked to this. Side-effects are rare but include nausea, vomiting, diarrhoea, fatigue, headache and there is increased risk of nephrotoxicity when used with nephrotoxic agents.[51] Current evidence is weak and not sufficient to justify its routine use.[52,53]

PHOTODYNAMIC THERAPY

Photodynamic therapy works on the principle of making specific target tissues susceptible to therapeutic intervention by prior administration of a photosensitive drug. The first drug used in RRP was dihaematoporphyrin ether (DHE). This compound has a propensity to concentrate within rapidly growing tissues such as papillomas rather than in surrounding normal tissue. Patients are typically treated intravenously with 4.25 mg/kg of DHE prior to surface treatment of papillomas by photo-activation with an argon pump dye laser. A small, but statistically significant, decrease in RRP growth has been noted and this effect is maximal in patients with aggressive disease and endobronchial lesions.[54] Generalised photosensitivity of the skin may occur as a side-effect of this therapy for between 2–8 weeks. Rarely, this may lead to cutaneous burns, which greatly reduces the potential use of this modality in children. Meso-tetra (hydroxyphenyl) chlorin has also been used and has shown efficacy in rabbits with minimal tissue damage and less photosensitivity. A randomised trial using a single episode of photodynamic therapy in 23 adults and children who had required surgery at least three times a year has been carried out; however, only 15 patients completed the trial.[55] Photodynamic therapy is available only in a small number of centres and current evidence is insufficient to justify its routine use.

INDOLE-3-CARBINOL

This is a dietary supplement derived from cruciferous vegetables (sprouts, broccoli, cabbage, cauliflower). It is thought to affect oestrogen metabolism, shifting production of oestrogen to an antiproliferative form.[56] It has been shown to affect *in vitro* papilloma growth.

It is administered orally at 100–200 mg in children weighing less than 25 kg.[54]

Its role in the management of JORRP remains uncertain. Studies have been non-randomised and with small numbers of patients. In a prospective observational study on a mixed adult and paediatric population, four of nine children who received indole-3-carbinol as an adjunct to surgical removal showed partial or total response with no evident side-effects.[57]

HEAT SHOCK PROTEINS (HSPS)

HspE7 is a recombinant fusion protein of Hsp56 from *Mycobacterium bovis* BCG and E7 protein from HPV 16. It has been administered subcutaneously to 27 children with JORRP.[58] Preliminary results suggested that HSP could prolong the interval between surgeries and reduce the number of procedures over a 60-week period. The effect was more marked in girls. The side-effects were mild-to-moderate local injection reactions. The authors suggested a Phase III trial on the basis of these encouraging results.

MUMPS VACCINE

The intralesional administration of mumps vaccine has been advocated as adjuvant therapy. The mechanism of action remains unclear but may relate to generalised stimulation of the host immune response. In a study of 29 children,[59] the mumps vaccine was administered at the time of surgical laser excision every 3–12 weeks with children receiving 1–26 injections with follow-up of 2–19 years. Twenty-three children were disease-free for at least one year and with two negative endoscopies. It is unclear how much of this was attributable to the variable natural history of the disease. Current evidence is insufficient to justify the routine use of mumps vaccine in JORRP.

CURRENT THERAPEUTIC STRATEGIES

Surgery remains the principal treatment modality for children with JORRP. Gastro-oesophageal reflux should be managed in accordance with local protocols. Of the available adjuvant therapies, cidofovir is the most immediately effective and, subject to the provisos above, should be considered for children who require multiple procedures or where tracheostomy seems imminent. Indole-3-carbinol has the merit of low toxicity but efficacy is uncertain. Interferon, acyclovir and ribavirin can only be recommended on an individual case basis if other modalities have failed. Photodynamic therapy is available in a limited number of centres but is largely impractical in children due to the persistence of cutaneous photosensitivity. HSP and mumps vaccine are currently under scrutiny.

HPV VACCINATION

Vaccines against HPV are now available. A quadrivalent vaccine containing antigenic material analogous to the L1 protein from the viral capsid of HPV subgroups 6, 11, 16 and 18 was licensed in the UK in September 2006.[60] There is some interest among otolaryngologists in the theoretical potential therapeutic effect of the quadrivalent vaccine for children with established JORRP, in whom it may act as a non-specific immunostimulant. The vaccine was developed for administration to young women where its primary role is in conferring immunity to the main causative agents of cervical uterine cancer (HPV 16 and HPV 18) and genital condylomata (HPV 6 and HPV 11). It is logical to expect that JORRP will be all-but eliminated if the quadrivalent vaccine is widely used, as looks likely at the time of going to press. The vaccine is particularly efficacious in girls aged 12–14 years. The cohort of girls now being offered HPV vaccination would be expected to have their first children in 5–10 years from now and it may be that JORRP will be virtually unknown in subsequent birth cohorts.

CONCLUSIONS

After much well-intentioned, but relatively poor quality, research there is a need for national or international registration of all RRP patients with exchange of data between centres. Well-designed, large, multicentre, randomised, controlled trials may establish the place of the various adjuvant treatments. Such is the rarity of this condition that international collaboration among specialist centres may be required to establish the optimum management of these patients. The potential for HPV vaccination to eliminate genital infection with HPV in young women may make JORRP almost unknown.

Key points for clinical practice

- Recurrent respiratory papillomatosis is known to be caused by the human papilloma virus.

- Tracheostomy should be avoided if at all possible given its potential to spread the disease.

- The microdebrider has now become the mainstay for most otolaryngologists in the treatment of recurrent respiratory papillomatosis.

Key points for clinical practice (continued)

- Advances in paediatric anaesthesiology and in peri-operative care of children has meant surgery for juvenile onset recurrent respiratory papillomatosis is increasingly done as a day case.

- Increasing centralisation should lead to better quality of care in this relatively uncommon condition.

- The evidence-base for most adjuvant treatments is poor.

- The decision to use cidofovir in recurrent respiratory papillomatosis should be taken cautiously and after discussion with the patient/parents about possible side-effects.

- Surgery is the mainstay of treatment and of the adjuvant therapies, cidofovir is considered by the authors to be the most effective.

- The licensing of vaccines against human papilloma virus may herald a decline in the rates of juvenile onset recurrent respiratory papillomatosis.

- Management in fewer centres should provide an easier means of undertaking larger scale trials of treatment regimens.

References

1. Shykhon M, Kuo M, Pearman K. Recurrent respiratory papillomatosis. *Clin Otol* 2002; **27**: 237–243.
2. Derkay CS, Darrow DH. Recurrent respiratory papillomatosis. *Ann Otol Rhinol Laryngol* 2006; **115**: 1–11.
3. Reidy PM, Dedo III I, Mathog RH *et al*. Integration of human papilloma virus type 11 in recurrent respiratory papilloma-associated cancer. *Laryngoscope* 2004; **114**: 1906–1909
4. Shah KV, Stern WF, Shah FK *et al*. Risk factors for juvenile onset recurrent respiratory papillomatosis. *Pediatr Infect Dis J* 1998; **17**: 372–376.
5. Derkay CS. Task force on recurrent respiratory papillomatosis. A preliminary report. *Arch Otolaryngol Head Neck Surg* 1995; **121**: 1386.
6. Lindeberg H, Elbrond O. Laryngeal papillomas: the epidemiology in a Danish subpopulation 1965–1984. *Clin Otolaryngol Allied Sci* 1991; **15**: 125–131.
7. Wiatrak BJ, Wiatrak DW, Broker TR, Lewis L. Recurrent respiratory papillomatosis: a longitudinal study comparing severity associated with human papilloma viral types 6 and 11 and other risk factors in a large pediatric population. *Laryngoscope* 2004; **114 (Suppl 104)**: 1–23.
8. Weiss MD, Kashima HK. Tracheal involvement in laryngeal papillomatosis. *Laryngoscope* 1983; **93**: 45–48.
9. Armstrong LR, Derkay CS, Reeves WC. Initial results from the National Registry for juvenile-onset Recurrent Respiratory Papillomatosis. *Arch Otolaryngol Head Neck Surg* 1999; **125**: 743–748.
10. Shapiro AM, Rimell FL, Shoemaker D *et al*. Tracheotomy in children with juvenile-onset recurrent respiratory papillomatosis: the Children's Hospital of Pittsburgh experience. *Ann Otol Rhinol Laryngol* 1996; **105**: 1–5.
11. Strong MS, Vaugh CW, Healy GB *et al*. Recurrent respiratory papillomatosis: management with a CO$_2$ laser. *Ann Otol Rhinol Laryngol* 1976; **85**: 508–516.
12. Tasca RA, McCormick M, Clarke RW. British Association of Paediatric Otorhinolaryngology members experience with recurrent respiratory papillomatosis

2006; *Int J Pediatr Otorhinolaryngol* **70**: 1183–1187.

13. Karamzadeh AM, Wong BJF, Crumley RL, Ahuja G. Lasers in pediatric airway surgery: current and future clinical applications. *Laser Surg Med* 2004; **35**: 128–134.

14. Deskin RW. Laser laryngoscopy for papilloma removal. In: Bailey BJ. (ed) *Atlas of Head and Neck Surgery Otolaryngology*. Philadelphia, PA: Lippincott-Raven, 1998; 237–245.

15. Abramson AL, Steinberg BM, Winkler B. Laryngeal papillomatosis: clinical, histopathologic, and molecular studies. *Laryngoscope* 1987; **97**: 678–685.

16. Setliff RC, Parsons DS. The 'hummer': new instrumentation for functional endoscopic sinus surgery. *Am J Rhinol* 1994; **8**: 275–278.

17. Christmas Jr DA, Krouse JH. Powered instrumentation in functional endoscopic sinus surgery. I: Surgical technique. *Ear Nose Throat J* 1996; **75**: 33–36, 39–40.

18. Patel RS, MacKenzie K. Powered laryngeal shavers and laryngeal papillomatosis: a preliminary report. *Clin Otol* 2000; **25**: 358–360.

19. El-Bitar MA, Zalzal GH. Powered instruments in the treatment of recurrent respiratory papillomatosis: an alternative to carbon dioxide laser. *Arch Otolaryngol Head Neck Surg* 2002; **128**: 425–428.

20. Patel N, Rowey M, Tunkel D. Treatment of recurrent respiratory papillomatosis in children with the microdebrider. *Ann Otol Rhinol Laryngol* 2003; **112**: 7–10.

21. Pasquale K, Wiatrak B, Wooley A, Lewis L. Microdebrider versus CO_2 laser removal of recurrent respiratory papillomatosis: a prospective analysis. *Laryngoscope* 2003; **113**: 139–143.

22. Schraff S, Derkay CS, Bourke B, Lawson L. American Society of Pediatric Otolaryngology members' experience with recurrent respiratory papillomatosis and the use of adjuvant therapy. *Arch Otolaryngol Head Neck Surg* 2004; **130**: 1039–1042.

23. Jaquet Y, Monnier P, Van Melle G, Ravussin P, Spahn DR, Chollet-Rivier M. Complications of different ventilation strategies in endoscopic laryngeal surgery: a 10-year review. *Anesthesiology* 2006; **104**: 52–59.

24. Bjornson CL, Klassen TP, Williamson J *et al.*; Pediatric Emergency Research Canada Network. A randomised trial of a single dose of oral dexamethasone for mild croup. *N Engl J Med* 2004; **351**: 1306–1313.

25. Russel K, Weibe N, Saenz A *et al.* Glucocorticoids for croup. Cochrane Database Syst Rev 2004; (1): CD001955.

26. Derkay CS, Hester RP, Burke B, Carron J, Lawson L. Analysis of a staging system for prediction of surgical interval in recurrent respiratory papillomatosis. *Int J Pediatr Otorhinolaryngol* 2003; **68**: 1493–1498.

27. Steinberg BM, Topp WC, Schneider PS, Abramson AL. Laryngeal papilloma virus infection during clinical remission. *N Engl J Med* 1983; **308**: 1261–1264.

28. Holland BW, Koufman JA, Postma GN *et al.* Laryngopharyngeal reflux and laryngeal web formation in patients with pediatric recurrent respiratory papillomas. *Laryngoscope* 2002; **112**: 1926–1929.

29. Harcourt JP, Worley G, Leighton SE. Cimetidine treatment for recurrent respiratory papillomatosis. *Int J Pediatr Otorhinolaryngol* 1999; **51**: 109–113.

30. Armbruster C. Novel treatments for recurrent respiratory papillomatosis. *Expert Opin Investig Drugs* 2002; **11**: 1139–1148.

31. Nodarse-Cuni H, Iznaga-Marin N, Viera-Alvarez D *et al.* Interferon alpha-2b as adjuvant treatment of recurrent respiratory papillomatosis in Cuba: National Programme (1994–1999 report). *J Laryngol Otol* 2004; **118**: 681–687.

32. Van Cutsem E, Snoeck R, Van Ranst M *et al.* Successful treatment of a squamous papilloma of the hypopharynx-esophagus by local injections of (S)-1-(3-hydroxy-2-phosphonylmethoxypropyl)cytosine. *J Med Virol* 1995; **45**: 230–235.

33. Pransky SM, Magit AE, Kearns DB *et al.* Intralesional cidofovir recurrent respiratory papillomatosis in children. *Arch Otolaryngol Head Neck Surg* 1999; **125**: 1143–1148.

34. Giles BL, Selfert B. Nebulised cidofovir for recurrent respiratory papillomatosis: a case report. *Paediatr Respir Rev* 2006; **7 (Suppl 1)**: S330.

35. Sheahan P, Sexton S, Russel JD. Is intralesional cidofovir worthwhile in juvenile recurrent respiratory papillomatosis? *J Laryngol Otol* 2006; **120**: 561–565.

36. Chetri DK, Shapiro NL. A scheduled protocol for the treatment of juvenile recurrent respiratory papillomatosis with intralesional cidofovir. *Arch Otolaryngol Head Neck Surg* 2003; **129**: 1081–1085.

37. Pransky SM, Albright JT, Magit AE. Long-term follow-up of pediatric recurrent respiratory papillomatosis managed with intralesional cidofovir. *Laryngoscope* 2003; **113**: 1583–1587.
38. Chung BJ, Akst LM, Koltai PJ. 3.5 year follow up of intralesional cidofovir protocol for pediatric recurrent respiratory papillomatosis. *Int J Pediatr Otorhinolaryngol* 2006; **70**: 1911–1917.
39. Naiman AN, Ceruse P, Coulombeau B *et al*. Intralesional cidofovir and surgical excision for laryngeal papillomatosis. *Laryngoscope* 2003; **113**: 2174–2181.
40. Derkay C. Cidofovir for recurrent respiratory papillomatosis (RRP): a re-assessment of risks. *Int J Pediatr Otorhinolaryngol* 2005; **69**: 1465–1467.
41. Lindsay F, Pransky S, Brewster D *et al*. Histologic review of cidofovir treated respiratory papillomatosis. Presented at American Branch Esophagologic Association, Phoenix, AZ, 30 April 2004.
42. Inglis AF. Cidofovir and the black box warning. *Ann Otol Rhinol Laryngol* 2005; **114**: 834–835.
43. Isaacs A, Lindenmann J. Virus interference I. The interferon. *J Proc R Soc Lond B Biol Sci* 1957; **147**: 258–267.
44. Haglund S, Lundquist PG, Cantell K, Strander H. Interferon therapy in juvenile laryngeal papillomatosis. *Arch Otolaryngol* 1981; **107**: 327–332.
45. Healy GB, Gelber RD, Trowbridge AL *et al*. Treatment of recurrent respiratory papillomatosis with human leukocyte interferon. Results of a randomised multicenter randomised clinical study. *N Engl J Med* 1988; **319**: 401–407.
46. Leventhal BG, Kashima HK, Mounts P *et al*.; Papilloma Study Group Long term response of recurrent respiratory papillomatosis to treatment with lymphoblastoid interferon alfa-N1. *N Engl J Med* 1991; **325**: 613–617.
47. Gerein V, Rastorguev E, Gerein J *et al*. Use of interferon-alpha in recurrent respiratory papillomatosis: 20 year follow up. *Ann Otol Rhinol Laryngol* 2005; **114**: 463–471.
48. Ventre K, Randolph AG. Ribavirin for respiratory syncytial virus infection of the lower respiratory tract in infants and young children. *Cochrane Database Syst Rev* 2006; CD000181.
49. McGlennen RC, Adams GL, Lewis CM *et al*. Pilot trial of ribavirin for the treatment of laryngeal papillomatosis. *Head Neck* 1993; **15**: 504–513.
50. Morrison GA, Kotecha B, Evans JN. Ribavirin treatment for juvenile respiratory papillomatosis. *J Laryngol Otol* 1993; **107**: 423–426.
51. Endres DR, Bauman NM, Burke D *et al*. Acyclovir in the treatment of recurrent respiratory papillomatosis. A pilot study. *Ann Otol Rhinol Laryngol* 1994; **103**: 301–305.
52. Kimberlin DW. Current status of antiviral therapy for juvenile-onset recurrent respiratory papillomatosis. *Antiviral Res* 2004; **63**: 141–151.
53. Morrison GA, Evans JN. Juvenile respiratory papillomatosis: acyclovir reassessed. *Int J Pediatr Otorhinolaryngol* 1993; **26**: 193–197.
54. Bauman NM, Smith RJ. Recurrent respiratory papillomatosis. *Pediatr Otolaryngol* 1996; **43**: 1385–1401.
55. Shikowitz MJ, Abramson AL, Steinberg BM *et al*. Clinical trial of photodynamic therapy with meso-tetra (hydroxyphenyl) chlorin for respiratory papillomatosis. *Arch Otolaryngol Head Neck Surg* 2005; **131**: 99–105.
56. Newfield L, Goldsmith A, Bradlow HL *et al*. Estrogen metabolism and human papillomavirus-induced tumours of the larynx: chemo-prophylaxis with indole-3-carbinol. *Anticancer Res* 1993; **13**: 337–341.
57. Rosen CA, Bryson PC. Indole-3-carbinol for recurrent respiratory papillomatosis: long-term results. *J Voice* 2004; **18**: 248–253.
58. Derkay CS, Smith RJH, McClay J *et al*. HspE7 treatment of pediatric recurrent papillomatosis: final results of an open-label trial. *Ann Otol Rhinol Laryngol* 2005; **114**: 730–737.
59. Pashley NR. Can mumps vaccine induce remission in recurrent respiratory papilloma? *Arch Otolaryngol Head Neck Surg* 2002; **128**: 783–786.
60. Vaccine to prevent cervical cancer and warts is licensed for use in the UK. *CDR Weekly* 2006; Vol 16.

Index

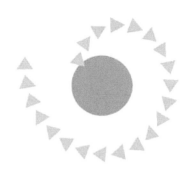

Acid monitoring 87–8
Acid-suppressive treatment 89–90
Acoustic neuroma 44–5
Acyclovir 164
Adrenaline 160
America Society of Pediatric Otolaryn-
    gology 160
American Academy of
    Otolaryngology–Head and Neck
    Surgery 148
American Joint Cancer Committee,
    TNM classification 68
Amitriptyline 150
Antibiotics against biofilms 28–9
Auditory brainstem implant 33–4
    ICC site 34–5
    patients benefitting 34
Auditory canal carcinoma with
    temporomandibular joint pain 71
Auditory midbrain implant 33–54
    clinical study 44
    description 36–7
    electrophysiological feasibility 37–40
    histomorphological effects 40–2
    psychophysical results 46–9
    speech results 49–51
    surgical approach 42–4
Auditory stimulation patterns 47–8

Bilitec 2000 88

Binaural intelligibility level difference 56
Binaural masking level difference 56
Biofilms 21–2
    bacterial
        aggregation 23–4
        attachment 22–3
        infections 21–31
        treatment strategies 28–9
    as bacterial reserve 25
    in chronic osteoradionecrosis 27–8
    development 22–4
    in infected cholesteatoma 26–7
    and middle ear implant infections 27
    in otitis media 25–6
    phenotype 23
    survival mechanisms 24–5

Cancer, immunotherapy 112
Carboplatin 125
Carotid invasion in temporal bone SCC 75
Cervarix 115
Cetuximab 130
Chemoradiotherapy 96, 122
    combination 125
    imaging after 127–8
    long-term sequelae 124
    new agents 130
    and organ preservation 123–4
    postoperative 126
Chemotherapy

combination 125
induction 128–30
temporal bone SCC 76
Cholesteatoma
    acquired 3
        MRI 9, 11, 13
    auto-evacuated 13
    congenital 1, 3, 5
    CT imaging 3–5
    infected, biofilms in 26–7
    MRI 1–20
        diffusion-weighted 5
    pars flaccida 3, 5
    pars tensa 3
    postoperative, MRI 13, 15, 17
    recurrent 3, 17
    signal intensity 7
    surgery 3
Cholesterol granuloma 9
Cidofovir 162–3, 165
Cisplatin+5-FU+taxane, trial results 129
Cisplatin
    cytotoxicity 124–5
    ototoxicity 124
Clarithromycin 29
Cochlear implantation
    bilateral 55–62
        after meningitis 58
        contraindications 59
        directional and spatial hearing
            establishment 57–8
        ethical, economic and legal
            considerations 59–60
        history 57
        improved speech understanding 57
        optimal time for 59
    simultaneous or sequential 58
    stimulation strategies 49
Cochlear implants 33
Computed tomography see CT
Computer-aided surgery 137
Consensus Conference on Cochlear
    Implants, 2nd, Valencia 60
Cranial nerve palsies 73
CT
    cholesteatoma 3–5
    intra-operative 143
    in rhinosinusitis 148
CT-MRI fusion 140–2

Deafness see Hearing loss
Dendritic cell based therapies 115–16
    in HNSCC 116
Dexamethasone 161
Diet change in GER 90
Dihaematoporphyrin ether 164
DNA
    microarray technologies 103–4
    mutations in HNSCC 95
Docetaxel 129
Duodenogastro-oesophageal reflux,
    non-acidic detection 88
Dural involvement in temporal bone
    SCC 75
Dysosmia 148

Electric currents against biofilms 28–9
Electrophoresis, two-dimensional gel
    97–8
Endoscopy 89
    nasal 148
    sinus surgery, CAS 137
Epidermal growth factor receptors 130
Epidermoid cyst 1
Epidermoid tumour 1
Epstein-Barr virus 116–18
    and nasopharyngeal carcinoma 117
Erythromycin 29
Eustachian tube
    functions 82–3
    reflux passage 84–5
Extra-oesophageal reflux
    interaction with OME 84–5
    in OME 80
Extra-oesophageal reflux disease
    definition 79
    diagnosis 86–7
    prevalence 80
    risk factors 82

Facial nerve 73
Facial pain 148–9
    midfacial segment 149–51
Fiducial localisation error 139
Fiducial registration error 139
Fiducials 138–40
Fluorodeoxyglucose-positron emission

tomography 128, 132
Fluoroscopy, intra-operative 143
Furanones 29

Gardasil 115
Gastric scintiscan 89
Gastro-oesophageal reflux, control of
    162, 165
Gastro-oesophageal reflux disease
    definition 79
    mechanism 81
    pathology 81
    prevalence 80
    risk factors 82
    symptoms 86
Gastro-oesophageal reflux
    disease/pharyngeal reflux,
    prevalence 83-4
Gene
    expression analysis 106
    multiple mutations 106
    targeted therapy 106
Gene Chip 103
Genetic material in biofilms 25
Genomics 103-6
Glucocorticoids 161

Head and neck cancer, vaccines and
    immunotherapy 111-20
Head and neck squamous cell carcinoma
    113
    chemotherapy 121-36
    meta analyses 129
    early diagnosis/screening 101-2
    metastasis prediction 105
    molecular classification 105-6
    prognosis and treatment response
        102-3
    progression prediction 104-5
    proteomics and genomics 95-109
    targeted management 106
Headache, tension-type 149-50
Hearing
    binaural 55-6
        auditory pattern recognition 56
        cocktail party phenomenon 56
        head shadow effect 56, 57

improved in noise 56
interaural level and time differences
    55-6
sound source location 56
spatial 55
Hearing loss
    long-term, effects 49
    sensorineural 124
Heat shock proteins 165
Hirsch's modified Pittsburgh Staging
    System 69
Hoarseness in JORRP 156
Human Genome Project 99
Human papilloma virus 113-15, 155-6
    carcinogenesis 114
    in HNSCC 95, 114
    vaccination 166
    vaccines in HNSCC 114-15
Hyperfractionation 126
Hyposmia 149

Ibuprofen 150
Image-guided surgery 137-46
    accuracy 137-40
    preoperative radiological data 138
    registration 142
    tracking systems 143
Immunotherapy
    definitions 112
    nasopharyngeal carcinoma 117-18
Implant, auditory midbrain 33-54
Indole-3-carbinol 165-6
Inferior colliculus 34-6
Interferon 163 4
International Society for Computer-
    Aided Surgery 137
Intra-operative localising device 143
Intraluminal impedance measurement 88
Iron salts 29
ISO 14155 44

Juvenile onset recurrent respiratory
    papillomatosis see Recurrent
    respiratory papillomatosis

Langerhans cells 115
Laryngopharyngeal reflux

pathological mechanisms 82
pH monitoring 87–8
Larynx
    examination 87
    in JORRP 156
Lip-reading 49–50
Loudness growth functions 48
Lymph node dissection, role 127

Magnetic resonance imaging *see* MRI
MALDI 99–100, 102
Mass spectrometry 98–9
Mastoidectomy and radiotherapy 71
Matrix-assisted laser desorption and
    ionization *see* MALDI
Medtronic electromagnetic system 143
Meningitis, bilateral cochlear
    implantation after 58
Meso-tetra chlorin 164
Middle ear
    epithelium injury 85
    implant infections, and biofilms 27
MRI
    cholesteatoma 1–20
        acquired 9, 11, 13
        congenital 7, 9
    diffusion-weighted 7, 15, 17
    echoplanar diffusion-weighted 17
    fast spin echo 7
    intra-operative 143
    late post-gadolinium T1-weighted
        imaging 13, 15, 18
    postoperative cholesteatoma 13, 15, 17
    primary bony obliteration techniques 18
    protocol 18
    turbo spin echo 7
Mucositis 123, 124, 125
Mumps vaccine 165

Nasopharyngeal carcinoma 117
    adoptive immunotherapies 118
    immunotherapy 117–18
Neck management 72
Neurofibromatosis type 2, ABI for 33–4

Oesophagus
    biopsy 89
    mucosal injury pathogenesis 81
    physiological protection 81

Osteoradionecrosis 131
    chronic, biofilms in 27–8
Otitis media
    biofilms in 25–6
    chronic suppurative, in SCC 63–4
    definition 80
    recurrences 24
    with reflux and effusion 79–93
Otitis media with effusion
    aetiology 82–3
    consequences 83
    definition 80
    diagnosis 86
    link with reflux 83–4
    pathogenesis 83
    patients at risk 83
    risk factors 83
Otology, bacterial biofilm infections in
    21–31

Paclitaxel 129
Papillomatosis
    recurrent respiratory
        adjuvant therapies 161–6
        anaesthesia 160
        care centralisation 161
        juvenile onset 156, 160–6
        laser surgery 158
        microdebrider 159–60
        peri-operative care 160–1
        surgery 157–61
        tracheostomy 160
        treatments 155–69
Paranasal sinus, CAS 137
Parotidectomy, superficial 71
Pepsin 81
    in OME 84–5
Pharyngeal acid reflux 84
Photodynamic therapy 164–5
Pittsburgh Staging System 69
Pituitary surgery, trans-sphenoidal,
    fusion technology 142
Planktonic cells, detachment and release
    24
Positron emission tomography 140
Post-transplant lymphoproliferative
    disease 118
Promotility agents 90
Protein profile of cancer cell 96–7

ProteinChip 100
Proteomes
    comparison 99
    description 96
Proteomics 96–103
    description 97
    expression 97–9
        profiling application 101–2
Proton pump inhibitors 89–90

Quorum sensing 23

Radiation Therapy Oncology Group 126, 127
Radiation-associated tumours 64–5, 76
Radiological information, intra-operative updating 142–3
Radiotherapy
    3-D conformal 130–1
    dose-fractionation studies 125–6
    intensity-modulated 131–2
    schedule improvement 125–6
Reflux
    acidic 81
    pH monitoring 87–8
    symptoms 85–6
Reflux-associated ear disorders 84
Rehabilitation after temporal bone SCC 74
Rhinosinusitis
    bacterial 148
    chronic
        diagnosis 148–9
        prevalence 147–53
Rhinosinusitis Task Force 148
Ribavirin 164

SELDI 100
Sinus infection, acute 150
Sinusitis, chronic 147
Skull base surgery, CAS 137
Soft tissue shift 143
Spatial hearing 55, 57
SPEAK strategy 40, 49
Spectral coding 48–9
Speech perception 48
Squamous cell carcinoma
    temporal bone 63–78
        aetiology 63–5

clinical symptoms 65
complications 73–4
diagnosis 66–7
epidemiology 65
histology 75
imaging 67–8
nodal disease 75
patterns of spread 66
presenting symptoms frequency 65
prognosis 74
radiotherapy 69–70
reconstruction 72–3
sleeve resection 70
staging 68–9
surgery 70–2, 75–6
survival related to TNM stage 74
Steroids 161
Stridor in JORRP 156
Surface enhanced laser desorption and ionization see SELDI
Surgeon-computer workstation interface 138

Target registration error 139
Taxanes 125, 132
Temporal bone
    extended resection 71
    lateral resection 70–1, 74
    squamous cell carcinoma 63–78
    subtotal resection 74
Toxico-genomics Research Consortium 105
Tracheostomy 156, 160
Transcriptome 97
Trigeminal caudal nucleus 150
Tumour vaccine, overview 112–13

UV light in SCC 63

VA Laryngeal Cancer Study 122
Vaccination
    history 111
    human papillomatosis virus 166
Vaccines
    HPV, in HNSCC 114–15
    mumps 165
    types 111–12
    see also Tumour vaccine

Weight reduction in GER 90